DATE DUE

MENTAL ILLNESS FOR CAREGIVERS

Irving G. Walmann

Alma Publishing, Gladstone, Missouri

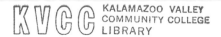

Mental Illness For Caregivers
by Irving G. Walmann

Published by: **ALMA Publishing**
Post Office Box 28268
Gladstone, MO 64188

Library of Congress Catalog Card Number: 98-70655

ISBN 0-9663299-5-3

Cover Illustration: Robert Howard

Publisher's Cataloging-in-Publication
(Provided by Quality Books, Inc.)

Walmann, Irving G.
 Mental illness for caregivers / Irving G, Walmann. -- 1st ed.
 p. cm.
 Includes bibliographical references and index.
 ISBN: 0-9663299-5-3

 1. Mental illness--Popular works. 2. Brain chemistry--Popular works. 3. Mental illness--Alternative treatment. 4. Pyruvic acid--Therapeutic use. I. Title.

RC460.W34 1998   616.85'2
                        QBI98-353

CONTENTS

LIST OF ILLUSTRATIONS

PROLOGUE

Because my own son became mentally ill at the age of seven, I've spent almost forty years reading about mental illness. During this time, I've looked for ways to help the mentally ill and ways to understand them. I feel that understanding those who are ill is important, because, if we don't understand, how can we relate? I've also given considerable thought to what I've read on the chemical workings of the brain, relative to mental illness --again, always looking for ways that the apparent chemical problems causing mental illness may be corrected.

The early reading I did fell into two parts: books by chemists, who tried to find body chemistry of the mentally ill which was different from the chemistry of others, and books by those who (like the ancient Greeks) tried to solve the problems of mental illness by thinking about them. The chemists were successful in producing the medications which are doing so much good in the treatment of mental patients, today. They were also successful, as far as I'm concerned, because they germinated the ideas which grew into this book. The efforts of the theorists, while controlling the practice of psychiatry for many of the ensuing years, have gradually given way to the efforts of the chemists, who today are almost in complete control of the situation.

That brings us to the reasons this book was

written. Through this book, I hope to accomplish several things--to help relatives and friends of those who are mentally ill to understand them better and those who are less ill to understand their own problems, to tell what has been done in the past and what is now being done to help them, to explain the causes of mental illnesses (as I see them), and to offer what I feel will be cures for many and preventions for most of these illnesses.

These are a great many things to try to accomplish with such a small book! But, I do hope to help the reader to understand the problems of the ill and the causes of mental illnesses, and I do offer what I hope will be cures and preventions. I say will be, because there is still testing to be done and probable genetic engineering to be done on bacteria.

Let's be frank about it--lots of wonderful work has been done, in learning how the brain works--and lots of wonderful work has been done, in treating the **symptoms** of mental illness--but not enough has been done to **cure and prevent** these problems. This book offers steps toward curing and preventing mental illness--now let's see who will take the ball and run with it!!

I hope I live to see all of these things come about, because, how could one ask more from one's life, than to bring pleasure to those who have had little pleasure, and to those who are yet unborn, through the elimination of mental illness.

ON CAREGIVING

I hope that many professional caregivers will read this book. But, caregivers also fall into many non-professional categories: brothers and sisters, parents, spouses, school teachers, friends, leaders of various organizations, and many others.

When our son was in school, now many years ago, his psychiatrists felt that his teachers should not be told of his problems, feeling that it was best for him to be treated in as close to a normal manner as possible. But there were times he was scolded by his teachers rather severely, when if the teachers had known of and understood his problems, he might have been treated more gently. Teachers, after all, have the same feelings of irritation as the rest of us, and probably have more offenders rubbing against those irritations than the rest of us. I think teachers are caregivers by nature--if they weren't, they wouldn't be teaching for a living--and I feel that our son's teachers, as caregivers, should have been told of his problems.

Although I feel that the psychiatrists may have been in error on that subject, I believe that psychiatrists, being those most able to help those we love, should be listened to and complied with. We shouldn't nullify their efforts by constantly trying to second-guess them. No, they aren't always right--who is?--but they are, at any given time, very close to the truth, as the truth is then known. (The accepted "truths" of mental illness have been revised many times, and I hope that this book will bring further revisions.) But back to caregiving.

It is, I think, especially important to inform brothers and sisters of a young person's mental problems, and also of a spouse's problems. Even small children will act differently toward one they know to be ill, and will try to understand. In families not plagued by mental illness, relationships between brothers and sisters are oftentimes full of stress. With mental illness, such relationships can become severely stressed. An open truthfulness can go far in relieving such stresses.

Very young children are capable, in my opinion, of understanding many things which are often considered understandable only by adults. And having worked with Cub Scout Webelos, I believe that, by the time young people reach the age of eleven, they are able to understand anything they will later understand as adults. They can be very capable caregivers.

Being a parent isn't an easy job at best, but the parents of those who are mentally ill are indeed hard pressed. Let's make no bones about it--the parents and spouses of the mentally ill have less fun in life than others. For the parents and spouses of the seriously mentally ill, caregiving oftentimes becomes a lifelong occupation--it has for my wife and myself.

Almost all people want similar things out of life: fun with our mates and children and friends; sexual fulfillment; to have children we can be proud of and brag about; and to pass our lineage on through healthy and bright children.

When our children or other loved-ones become seriously mentally ill, we still love them and wish them well, but we know in our hearts that they don't stand a snowball's chance of having a happy life--the more serious the mental problems, the less happy their life is likely to be. And yet, we try to help them, and to understand them (our children, our spouse, or parent, or...), and it's only natural to try to figure out how life could have done us such a dirty trick.

So many of us, oftentimes without our choice, become caregivers. We would much rather that our children, our brothers and sisters, our parents and friends, had been mentally completely normal. But here we are, regardless of our choice, caregivers. And, let's face it-- how many would choose to be care-receivers, instead?

The honest truth is that none of us would want to be in their shoes. We want to help them, we want to do everything we can to help them, but we don't want to be mentally ill. That's normal and proper. If we were seriously ill, too, how could we help them?

Besides, though it sounds like a trite thing to say, the truth is that we're caregivers because we do care. In the same way, I believe that most doctors, nurses and social workers are doing the work they do because deep-down they care, too. They care a great deal, I'm sure. There may be many people who care about the mentally ill, more than they usually say.

So, we want to know what we can do to help those we know who are mentally ill. It seems that the only things possible to do, so far, have been to treat them with kindness and to get for them what help is medically available.

Through this book, we can go two steps further--we can gain an understanding of the problems with which they are struggling--and, by giving this book to our medical acquaintances, we may be able to eventually bring further help to them, and help prevent illness in others, in the future.

Ch 1
MENTAL ILLNESS - THE PROBLEM
AND THE PROMISE

Life is hard. Oh, life can be very pleasant, too--but for those who are mentally ill, life is almost always hard. How many people are we talking about? Well, of all those who go to medical doctors, 21.7% go for mental or addictive problems (16% of the people of the United States)[1]. In our country (which is surely not so different from the rest of the world), about twenty percent (one in five) of all women will seek medical help for depressive illness at some time in their lives. And, while a smaller percentage of men are diagnosed with depressive illness, most of those who commit suicide because of it are male.

The number of people who kill themselves because of depressive illness each year, in our country alone, is about 30,000[2] (and how many more attempt suicide, or feel very close to it?). Teenagers are particularly vulnerable, because the teen years can be trying enough without mental illness. When depressive illness is added, things can get beyond one's ability to handle, and suicide may seem the only way out.

Another two percent of the world's people have schizophrenia--over a hundred-million people world-wide. It has been said that schizophrenia is far worse than cancer. I don't know whether that is true or not, but since our oldest son (now forty-six) has schizophrenia, I do know from firsthand experience that--even with the medications now available--it is never easy or fun.

There are many other mental illnesses, some of which are discussed in chapter four. In the United States, each year, about fifteen percent of adults receive mental health services of some sort[3]. Of those in need of such services, one-fifth go to mental health specialists, three-fifths to general practitioners (GPs), and the other fifth go untreated[4]. The salary totals for those whose work is treating the mentally ill exceed fifty billion dollars a year in our country, and when you add in the cost of hospitals and housing, the total cost is over 150 billion dollars each year[5]. But it's tough getting millions, or even thousands, for research.

Depressive illness in the United States costs over forty-four billion dollars each year in treatment and wages lost. And that's not the most important thing. Suicides among teenagers and young adults are on the increase, and three percent of all Americans will attempt suicide at some time. Clearly, something needs to be done now. That's said to be more easily said than done. I disagree...

The title of this chapter speaks of a promise. Yes, there is a promise here. I hesitate to make it, because many will think it impossible to fulfill--and therefore, will think me very foolish. I promise that before you reach the end of this book you will have learned the probable causes of both the depressive illnesses and schizophrenia--and you will have learned how, according to my findings, both of those problems can be eliminated.

So, I'll tell you in this book what I find to be the causes of these illnesses and how these problems can be corrected. If you want to, you can skip to about the middle of the book and find out what those causes are and what can be done about them. However, this isn't a long book and I've tried to write it in a manner that isn't too hard to read. I hope you'll stay with me, so that you'll come to know and understand what mental illness is all about. It may help those who are ill if we just understand, a bit better.

But, those who are influential in the science of the mind and in psychiatric medicine, as well as our own M.D.s, also need to read this book. That's where you, the reader, come in. If you become convinced that the ideas presented here are worthwhile, and if enough of you can get your medical friends to read this book, it may be that the suffering of the mentally ill can--in our lifetimes--finally come to an end.

Fig. 1. A rough idea of some brain duties.

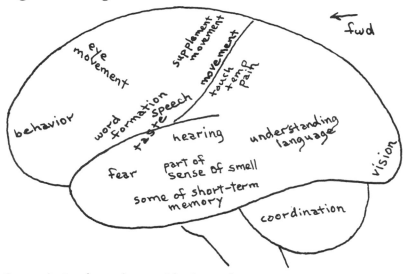

Some duties from the outside, inward.

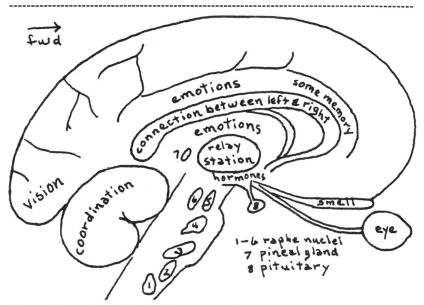

Some duties from the inside, outward.

Ch 2

HOW THE BRAIN WORKS

Though scientists, especially in the last fifty years, have made large advances in the treatment of the symptoms of mental illness and in the study of brain functions, it hasn't been easy--mostly because of the complexity of the brain. But because of their work, it's now possible for all of us to have an elementary understanding of the brain's workings.

First of all, it will help that understanding to hear some of the latest concepts on how the brain does the things it does--a subject on which the most expert of experts don't have a complete grasp, or agreement. Like the electronics field, it's an area where knowledge has been increasing very rapidly--and many rigidly-held ideas have had to give way.

I'd like to offer encouragement to those readers who are interested in the mentally ill, but who have had little training in science--particularly in the biological sciences. Please don't be overly concerned if my attempts in this chapter to explain the workings of the brain seem a little overwhelming. It is difficult to explain complex concepts in a simple manner--and the human brain is as complex a thing as exists. But this should be offset by the fact that it isn't necessary to understand each and every statement made here--there won't be a test afterward.

Let's start by saying that you're standing at the side of a street in a large city. Let's say that you just happen to be looking at a signboard across the street, and on the signboard are some printed words, a tiger, and (as unlikely as it seems) a cow. A car is moving along the street in front of you.

You're looking at the signboard with your eyes, of which the retinas, at least, are considered part of the brain. But the mind actually "sees" what you're looking at at the rear of the brain (to where the optic nerves and their continuations, the optic "tracts," take the visual information. Information also goes to the hypothalamus, the pineal gland and the brain stem, but let's not get too fancy, for the moment.).

To help you to be aware of and interpret the things you're seeing, the brain provides information from many other areas of the cortex (the "higher" areas of the brain)--these areas being at greater or lesser distances from the visual area (in the rear). Other parts of the brain provide other services.

As you read the words on the signboard, they're recognized by an area on the left side of your brain. If you should mumble the words to yourself, that's handled by another area on the left side. If the words arouse emotional feelings in you, that's probably handled by areas deep inside the brain and further processed on the right. Areas inward from your ears are involved in your short-term memory of the words (long-term memory seems to be wide-spread), and visual memory may be located near the vision areas (at the rear). If there is any three-dimensional effect on the sign, that's handled by the right side of your brain.

Looking at the tiger and the cow on the signboard, your recognition of them is probably aided by two other areas (one for domestic animals, perhaps, and another for "wild" animals). If you think about the names of the animals, that's probably handled by the same area that handled the printed words, but not necessarily.

The sounds you hear (and any odors you may smell) are processed by areas near your ears (the odors are helped by other areas, as well). If you recognize (with another area) the driver of the car going by as someone you dislike, and are tempted to say something unpleasant to him but think better of it, that self-control is probably handled behind your forehead. If the driver of the car says something sarcastic to you, the left side of your brain recognizes the words and the right side catches the sarcasm.

The colors and shapes of the sign and the car, as well as the speed and direction of the car's movement, are handled by areas immediately forward of the primary visual area at the rear and get their information directly from it[1]. The make and model of the car is categorized and possibly recognized by other areas. In looking at this scene, many other parts of the brain are also at work-- and, isn't the cooperation beautiful?!

During the above actions, millions of neurons (at least) have been at work--perhaps over half the neurons of the cortex (that "higher" area--the convoluted outer surface of the brain) taking some part. That's speaking of some billions of cells--and this doesn't mention the many millions of other cells which have been working away, carrying on the ordinary business of the brain--things like maintaining body temperature, blood pressure, hormone outputs, muscle control of balance and movement, etc.

Brain scientists feel that most of the other business of the brain may be being handled in much the same manner as vision--with information from a multitude of areas feeding into each area of action, and with each of these inputs having a chance to influence the results.

With this much insight into the overall operation of the brain, let's take a peek at the nuts and bolts.

Both the rigid structures of the body and the soft tissues are composed of **cells** (and fluids, of course). The brain, like the rest of the body, is made up of such cells. These cells are similar to bacteria (germs), but they're much more organized.

The cells of the brain come in many shapes and sizes (all very tiny), and have many functions. The cells we usually think of, when and if we think of the brain, are the neurons. They do the work of the brain, and one thing which makes the study of them particularly difficult is their sheer number.

There are estimated to be a hundred billion neurons in a human brain. And each of them has about a thousand nursemaid cells--which cushion them, insulate them electrically, take up unnecessary substances from around them, perhaps supply them with other substances, act as the "blood-brain barrier," (which keeps any potentially harmful substances in the blood from reaching the neurons) and (some suggest) may even act as storehouses for memory.

As if that weren't enough, each average neuron has a couple of thousand connections to other neurons, connections called **synapses**. The messages received by a neuron from other neurons come through such connections, most of them on thin out-branchings of the neuron, called **dendrites**. These (input message) dendrites look much like the fine roots of a plant, in super-miniature (See fig. 2, on the next page).

The messages passed onward by each neuron to other neurons are carried by a single larger root-like projection, which comes out of the main body of the neuron. It resembles the tap root of a tree, and is called an **axon**. This (outflow message) axon usually has a system of roots of its own at the end, with connections to many other neurons similar to those on the dendrites.

Each of these connections (both input and output synapses) receives most of its nutrients, and the materials from which to manufacture substances it needs, from the main body of the neuron, through those incredibly small root-like axon and dendrites, moving along phenomenally smaller tubes. Vesicles--tiny bubble-like spheres filled with needed materials--travel along the **outside** of these tubes, out through the axons and dendrites, to the synapses and other places where they are needed. Other vesicles go the other way, back to the main body of the neuron.

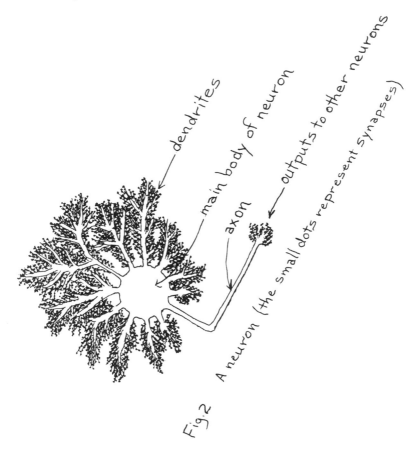

Fig. 2

A neuron (the small dots represent synapses)

dendrites

main body of neuron

axon

outputs to other neurons

Let's consider, for a moment, how many of the little chemical plants (connections/synapses) the brain operates. I'm no astronomer, but I do know that the milky way--that streak of stars we see across the night sky--is a portion of our own galaxy, the Milky Way Galaxy. Our galaxy is estimated to contain a hundred billions of stars (the same number as there are neurons in a human brain). And yet the number of synapses in a single human brain may approach the number of stars in two-thousand galaxies like our Milky Way.

Those synapses between neurons--the trillions of places where information is passed from one neuron to another--don't actually touch. There is about an 80 nanometer space (.00008 of a millimeter/.000003 of an inch) between the two sides of the synapse. In this space is a mat of protein fiber, which allows the passage of the transmitter (and other) chemicals, as well as acting to hold the two sides of the synapse in position, relative to each other[2]. When the upstream neuron "fires," it puts out one or more kinds of chemicals into this space, which the downstream neuron recognizes as signals and acts on those signals. The brain may use as many as a hundred different chemicals to pass these messages, and it's now thought that a single neuron may use several of them.

These chemicals released into the synapses to pass messages are called **transmitters**, like radio transmitters, and **neuropeptides**. Each synapse stores its transmitter molecules in tiny vesicles, similar to those mentioned above, from which they are released into the synaptic space (See figs. 3 and 4).

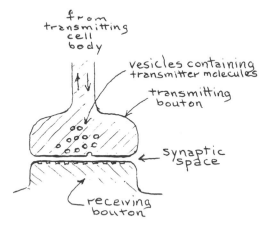

Fig. 3 A synapse -- approximate magnification 16,000 (based on synaptic space)

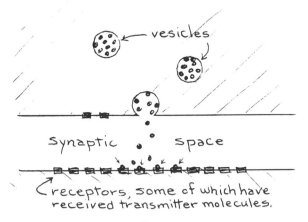

Fig. 4 Release of transmitter -- approx. mag. 190,000 (b.o.s.s.)

The two sides of each synapse apparently looked much like buttons to some researcher along the way. As a result, they were given the name of the French word for buttons--**boutons**. The two boutons of each synapse (one on the transmitting cell, and one on the receiving cell) can look like two incredibly tiny suction cups facing each other, except that, instead of the ends of the suction cups being concave (indented), they're both more or less flat. The transmitting bouton is somewhat-covered and the receiving bouton well-covered with **receptors**, which receive the transmissions of the upstream cell's transmitter chemicals. While the spaces between these surfaces are very small, they are very important, because they are the spaces through which the chemical messages pass.

The messages, to and from other neurons, have a variety of purposes. They can make the downstream neurons more likely to "fire" (that is, to send a message), they can make them less likely to fire, or they can bring about chemical reactions in the downstream neurons for other purposes.

Unfortunately for those who study the brain, the connections between neurons, while producing wonderful results and therefore presumably wonderfully well organized, don't seem at first glance to be well organized at all. Instead of a message passing in a "reasonable" manner from neuron A to neuron B to neuron C, etc., a single neuron, besides receiving connections (with messages) from thousands of other neurons, and putting out connections (with a message or messages) to a multitude of other neurons--oftentimes sends messages back to its own input, in what's called a feedback. Like the connections to other neurons, these feedback connections can make the neuron (itself) more or less likely to fire again.

With the transfer of needed substances from the blood of the brain to the cell bodies of the neurons--and then out along those tiny tubes to that astronomical number of synapses--and then, within those synapses, the manufacture of other needed substances--there's quite a shipping and manufacturing operation going on in each of our brains. And this doesn't even consider the tremendous manufacturing activity going on in the main bodies of the neurons themselves.

In summary, most of the connections bringing information into the neuron are attached to the (multiple root-like) dendrites, and the output information of the cell is sent by way of the single axon, which has multiple branches at the far end with connections to other neurons.

Considering the tremendous number of neurons, sending and receiving their messages by way of the astronomical number of synapses, the surprise may be that there aren't more mental problems than there are, since there are so many places for things to go wrong. Probably, there isn't any such surprise. It's quite likely that we have lots of glitches in our brains, but they just aren't serious enough to prevent our living a reasonably normal existence.

All of these complexities make the study of the

brain difficult. And, although a brain surgeon can take a moment to check something on the brain, one can't (in our society) examine the brain of a living person minutely. Unfortunately, examining the brains of cadavers leaves much to be desired, because of the changes that occur after death. Several pieces of equipment have been developed, however, which can provide considerable information from the outside (some of these will be briefly described in chapter three), and many procedures have been worked out that allow study in the lab.

There are some simplifying factors. The brain is anything but a random pile of billions of cells connected in a random manner. It's extremely well organized. And there are large groups of neurons working together to perform each job. This is fortunate, because the loss of a few cells isn't usually noticeable--Parkinson's disease, for instance, doesn't produce symptoms until most of the cells involved are no longer functioning.

How most of the messages transmitted by neurons accomplish the wonderful things the brain does is yet to be learned, but the messages of the transmitter **serotonin** are somewhat understood. Serotonin is made, in the synapses of neurons, from the amino acid tryptophan (one of the building blocks of proteins), and is important in depressive illness. It's probably also important in schizophrenia. Most of the time, serotonin works as an **inhibitor**; it tends to cause cells not to fire. When serotonin is in short supply, the downstream cells tend to be overactive, and that's a big part of the problem in much mental illness.

Fig. 5. EEG (electroencephalography).

My own rendition of a small part of an electroencephalogram readout (discussed in the next chapter):

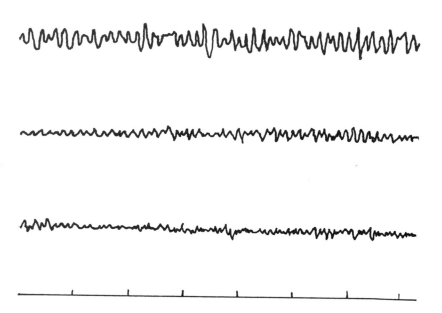

One can well-imagine that it took many such read-
outs, using subjects with known problems, before those
"squiggles" began to tell their stories.

Ch 3
MACHINES USED TO CHECK MENTAL
PROBLEMS AND TO STUDY THE BRAIN

There are quite a few machines in use to diagnose mental problems, get a view of shapes and forms in the brain, and to learn what's going on and where. These machines are referred to primarily by their abbreviations, such as EEG, CT, MRI, PET and SPECT. While of considerable use to doctors and of great use to brain scientists, and while these machines have revealed changes to the brain that occur with various mental problems, they aren't completely pertinent to the purpose of this book, so I'll give them only a summary treatment.

The **EEG** or **electroencephalogram**, which came into use about 1930, operates by detecting tiny electrical fields coming from various areas of the brain, amplifying them about a million times, and making those results visible as waves in continuous ink lines on a moving sheet of paper.

The use of EEGs has shown that there are many standard wave patterns emanating from various areas of the brain. The shapes of those waves depend on whether the subject has his or her eyes closed or open (and on what is seen), whether that person is awake or asleep (and how deeply asleep, if asleep), and other factors. Various mental illnesses can produce abnormal patterns, and lesions (injuries) to the brain can produce others. Epileptic seizures make striking patterns, abnormal metabolic problems (like the poor use of energy or of various substances by brain cells) produce other patterns. Those who record and interpret these patterns can often provide doctors with information not readily available through other means.

Another machine with which everyone is familiar is the **X-ray**. As far as the brain is concerned, the x-ray is used primarily to help determine the extent of accident injury, and may be used to locate and study tumors.

The **CT** or **computed axial tomography**, commonly called the "cat scan," uses a wonderful machine for checking the entire body. For brain purposes, it's especially useful in locating tumors and hemorrhages. Thousands of short bursts of x-rays are delivered, while the machine circles the body. A computer delivers a view to a TV screen of the internal structures, and an entire scanning delivers only a relatively small amount of x-ray radiation.

The **PET**, or **positron-emission tomography**, uses a short-lived radioisotope of oxygen (which, being radioactive, breaks up after only about two minutes) or a radioactive glucose (a short-lasting form of sugar). These substances are injected into the bloodstream and are carried by the blood to the brain. The breakdown emissions from them are detected, which either tell of the increased blood flow when part of the brain is in use, or tell of glucose (sugar) use.

The PET has been of great help in mapping brain areas active during specific brain activities, and shows areas as small as five millimeters (a quarter-inch). The brain areas active during the use of vision (discussed in chapter two), have been clearly shown in this manner. PET has the shortcomings of being expensive to operate and, because of the short life of the radioactive materials, having to be located right where those materials are made. So the PET is used primarily in research centers.

The **SPECT**, or **single photon emission computed tomography**, also uses radioactive materials--usually radioactive iodine or technetium--and, like the PET, works by viewing areas of greater blood flow. Its resolution is about 12 millimeters, showing things down to half an inch--with less than half the resolution of the PET.

Because the SPECT uses radioactive substances with longer lives than the PET uses, it can be located away from a cyclotron and is available in almost all clinical nuclear medicine facilities.

The **MRI**, or **magnetic resonance imaging** has the advantage of putting out no x-ray radiation and no radiation from radioactive dyes, and is said to have no known adverse effects. The patient is placed in a cylinder which is surrounded by a powerful magnet. Radio waves are then administered, and the atoms of the body "resonate" to the frequencies applied and put out their own radio waves, which, thru the use of computers, are pictured. The MRI produces images on a TV screen similar to those of the cat scan, but gives a much greater contrast between normal and abnormal tissues. It's particularly useful when dealing with soft tissues like the brain and spinal cord and has such a fine resolution that in the laboratory it's used in the study of molecules.

The cat scan and MRI work best for structural viewing, to see what things look like; the PET and SPECT are best for functional viewing, to see how well things are working.

Ch 4

SYMPTOMS OF MENTAL ILLNESS

I hope that none of you, reading this chapter, will come down with "medical student's disease" and decide that you have one or all of the following problems. However, if you seriously feel that you have one or more symptoms, you're not alone--millions of people do have them--and I urge you to discuss such symptoms with a physician. Most mental problems are handled, these days, by family physicians. They're quite capable of making judgements and prescribing medications, and will recommend a specialist should you need one. Proper medications can go a long way toward making a mental patient feel comfortable; the doctor's assurance that he doesn't need the medications may make him feel even more comfortable.

Please don't think that mental illness is a rare thing, or that people who have mental problems are peculiar--the unfortunate fact is that, unless cures for mental illnesses are found and used, some mental illness will affect about half the people of our country, to some extent, at some time in their lives.

No one can look at another person and know the thoughts and inner feelings that person is experiencing. So, to get an idea of what mental illness is like, one must go to the reports of doctors, who, in turn, use the words of their patients and the information they get from relatives of patients to make decisions. They also look for appearances and actions. When all is said and done, that's all even such worthy publications as the DSM IV (the diagnostic manual of the American Psychiatric Assn.) is able to offer. The physician has an additional tool--he can note the response to medications, both past and present. Let's take a look at some symptoms:

Depressive illness is an all-inclusive term which covers several closely-related illnesses--**major depression, psychotic depression, atypical depression and bipolar** (manic-depressive) **disorder**. These divisions aren't cut and dried; they have many variations. Perhaps the most important task of the doctor who treats depressive illness is to decide which of the variations of depressive illness the patient has, since the medication recommended for each of them is somewhat different (see chapter six for more about medications).

The first kind of depression I'll describe is MAJOR DEPRESSION, but I'd like to give a note of explanation first. The term "major depression" doesn't mean that the person has a bad case, or that this kind of depression is worse than other kinds; it's just a name. It's probable that many a person has been frightened by being told they had "major depression." If I were asked,

I'd suggest that the name be changed to "simple depression."

The person with **major depression** alternates between times of normalcy and times of deep depression. During the periods of depression, the person may lose interest in everything; may have feelings of being worthless; may have difficulty in "thinking;" may have changes in sleep patterns; may tire easily; may have a loss of appetite with a loss of weight; and/or have other symptoms. Perhaps the most distinguishing feature of major depression is that not even the most pleasant circumstance can bring a smile to the person's face. The worst time of the day is in the morning. The most worrisome symptom the person with major depression may have is thoughts of suicide. I've kept repeating the word "may," because a person with depressive illness may not have all of these symptoms. This is true of all mental illnesses, and is part of what makes choosing correct medications so difficult.

A person with **PSYCHOTIC DEPRESSION** has the symptoms of major depression, with added problems of a type usually associated with schizophrenia: having delusions and/or hallucinations. While the person with major depression may think she's bad and may think she deserves to die (twice as many women as men suffer with depressive illness), the person with psychotic depressive illness may hear a voice telling her how bad she is, and much less often may even see a person who's not there telling her these things. All of the delusions and hallucinations of the person with psychotic depression are self-deprecating or belittling in nature.

The name **ATYPICAL DEPRESSION** doesn't suggest that the problem isn't common (because it is), but merely that some of the symptoms are different from those of major depression.

One difference is that the patient can be cheered up, temporarily. And while the person with major depression may not get enough sleep, the person with atypical depression may be hard to get out of bed. While the major depressive may eat little and lose weight, the atypical depressive may overeat and gain weight. Any criticism is devastating. One feels worst in the evening.

One percent of the population have **BIPOLAR DISORDER** (MANIC-DEPRESSIVE ILLNESS). This amounts to about two and a half million people in our country alone.

Bipolar Disorder differs from Major Depression in that--in addition to times when one feels normal--periods of deep depression are alternated with what are called "manic" periods, during which one feels able to do **anything**. It's interesting that some of those who have this problem are successful in their fields (among them may have been several of our most famous writers and composers, whose names you may learn by checking the referred book, if you wish)[1], and many of their accomplishments have been made during their manic phases. This is so much true that some writers, artists and others discontinue their medications and suffer through the depressive phases, in order to have the creative highs of the manic phases[2]. That might be all right, except for the large numbers of bipolar

patients who commit suicide during their depressive phases. Before the 1970s, when lithium came into use as a
medication, twenty percent of those with bipolar
disorder died by suicide[3].

Very likely, before a doctor will state that his or
her patient has a depressive illness, symptoms will have
had to be present for a given length of time, such as two
weeks--but the expression of thoughts of suicide are
taken seriously immediately. Unfortunately, it's still true
that between sixty and eighty percent of the young
people who commit suicide have had a history of either
bipolar or major depression[4], and the rest must surely
have had one of the depressions.

In addition to the famous people who suffered
from bipolar depression, there have been successful and
even famous people who suffered from major (simple)
depressive illness--the most-often mentioned being
Abraham Lincoln--but most of them would have been
overjoyed to rid themselves of the problem. Perhaps this
can soon be accomplished, in all types of depressive
illness, by making a small increase in the amount of tryptophan reaching the brain (as discussed in later chapters).

SCHIZOPHRENIA is, at one and the same time,
one of the most common and most misunderstood illnesses. Two percent of the people of this earth have
schizophrenia (five million people in our country alone).
Because schizophrenia has so many different symptoms
and outcomes, it's thought by many experts to be a
collection of problems[5].

Many of us have accepted an old concept that a

person with schizophrenia has multiple personalities, but it just isn't so. (There is an increasingly diagnosed multiple-personality problem called DID or MPD--Dissociative Identity Disorder or Multiple Personality Disorder--which is sometimes diagnosed as schizophrenia, but is thought to be brought on by severe stress and seems to be distinct from schizophrenia.)

The most common symptom of schizophrenia is that of hearing a voice or voices. A voice out of nowhere may be berating the person for one thing or another (this will happen more or less frequently, depending on the severity of the illness). Two or more voices may hold a conversation, derisive of the person, in the background of the person's mind, or take turns commenting on every thought and action of the sufferer. (You can understand how difficult it is for these people to hold a normal conversation, if you consider how hard it would be for you to hold a telephone conversation with other people talking to you, every few seconds.)

The sufferer may have "delusions," and be **certain** that what he imagines to be true **is** true, when "ordinary" common sense tells the rest of us that these things simply can't be so. He or she, for instance, can't be talked out of the idea that some famous person came in, during the night, and stole something out of the closet.

Hallucinations are also a common phenomenon. While we usually think of hallucinations as visual, they can happen in any of the senses. The sufferer may see, smell, taste, feel or hear things that aren't really there. (It's my personal opinion, at least when the problem is visual, that the brain makes use of part of its normal visual apparatus to actually see hallucinations--perhaps drawing things out of visual memory--in some sort of faulty feedback. While I'm guessing, I'll guess that the brain may use memories in the other senses for the other types of hallucinations, as well.)

Most of those with schizophrenia lose their ability to plan for the future, and their drive to do anything. Happily, many of the symptoms of schizophrenia can be much lessened by medications. These make the patient much more comfortable, but usually leave him or her still unable to work at anything outside of very simple tasks.

People with schizophrenia may also have other problems of thought and behavior, but these are beyond the purpose of this chapter--which is to give the average person a feeling for the things the ill person has to live with, and a sense of urgency that these things must be cured.

ANXIETY DISORDERS are very common. They bring doctors their greatest number of mental patients. Perhaps five percent of the population suffer with anxiety problems which ought to be treated.

But anxiety can be normal and sometimes very useful. It's what would make you jump out of the way of a runaway truck, or fall to the floor when the bankrobber pulled a gun. It's what I felt when the doctor told me that I was either going to have a balloon procedure or a heart bypass operation.

Since the atomic bomb was discovered, and especially in our larger cities--where crime is considered almost normal--the "normal" anxiety level of our people has been on a steady increase and is taking a heavy toll in blood pressure and heart problems, and may be a factor in anxiety disorders. (I can't help noticing, when I visit New York City, that many men speak with voices more tenor than bass-- and speak much more rapidly--than I think they would if they lived in some other part of the country. I'll grant, though, that this may be a matter of local custom, rather than of anxiety.)

Generalized Anxiety Disorder (GAD) is a constant and exaggerated form of anxiety. People with GAD tend to be always tired, have trouble at work and are at greater than normal risk of getting hooked on alcohol, trying to escape the anxiety. Fortunately, there are several drugs which are effective in relieving the problem.

A **Panic Attack** starts with a sudden increase in anxiety. Your heart pounds and hands shake, you may have trouble breathing, may feel dizzy and may start sweating. There are quite a few other feelings you may have. You know that something is very wrong and don't know what it is--but whatever it is, it's extremely fright- ening. By the time you get to a hospital, everything can be back to normal. The emergency room doctor may not find a thing wrong--but that doesn't stop you from being terribly afraid that an attack will happen again.

Panic attacks can happen repeatedly, but even if it happens only once, it's so frightening that you can become more and more anxious about the next attack. **Phobias**, fear of harmless things like birds, cats or garter snakes can develop if you see such things during an attack. Even your increased breathing rate, perspiration and faster heartbeat during sex may remind you of a panic attack--make you think it's happening again, and cause you to be afraid to continue.

It's typical that the thought of the embarrassment and humiliation of being seen during a panic attack can make you stay away from more and more places. Finally, you may become so anxious and worried that you make great changes in your life style, so as to be able to get to a hospital as quickly as possible if it happens again. Most everything gets cancelled, so you will be ready (and alone or with only a close confidant) if it happens. The great anxiety which causes one to do these things is what's referred to as **Panic Disorder**. OCD (obsessive-compulsive disorder--see below) can evolve, too, with the idea developing that if you do this or that repeatedly, you can avoid another panic attack.

About 1.3% of the population have a panic disorder in any given year[6], and perhaps 2% get one at some time in their lives. It's interesting that many of the drugs effective in preventing panic attacks are also effective antidepressants, and it may be that an increase in brain tryptophan level would eliminate panic disorders (this is discussed in later chapters). It's fortunate that medications do work, because panic disorder (and similar problems) literally do disorder one's entire life.

Obsessive Compulsive Disorder (OCD) is also considered an anxiety problem. It involves compulsive thoughts and/or actions, such as wondering over and over again, endlessly, whether you locked the doors when you left the house, or (when you're home) actually checking the locks (or washing your hands), over and over and over. If the thought or action is resisted, anxiety builds up and up, until one feels forced to release the anxiety by thinking the thought or taking the action. About two percent of the population are said to have this problem[7]. (Since OCD is treated with antidepressants, it too might yield to an increase in brain tryptophan level.)

BORDERLINE PERSONALITY DISORDER takes another two percent of the population. These folks suffer from an extreme fear of rejection from friends, relatives and even caregivers. They're very impulsive in spending their money, driving their car, or in whatever they're doing. They may alternate between loving and hating a person. There many be even less-desirable characteristics, including tendencies toward self-mutilation and suicide.

Many of these most common mental disorders can be much improved through medication, allowing those with lesser problems to lead lives almost free of excess mental distractions and to continue in their former employment. Oftentimes, even those with more severe illness are able to work in "workshops" set up especially for them and supported by good businesses, to gain the sufferers a little spending money.

Ch 5

PAST AND PRESENT TREATMENT
OF MENTAL PROBLEMS

First, a little ancient history. To begin with, I imagine that there have been mental problems as long as there has been man. But in the really early days, when one was probably trying to stay a few steps ahead of the predators, those who were mentally ill no doubt had a short life expectancy.

The earliest treatment of mental illness may have been found in ancient skulls from the Neolithic Age, which had quite skillful trepanning (or trephining)--holes made in the skulls--as if modern brain surgery had been done. It's felt that the holes were made to let evil spirits out--the evil spirits of mental illness-- although we don't know that they weren't done to correct severe injury to the skull. That the trepanning was skillfully done is evident, because the patients lived, as indicated by the fact that the bone of the skulls had healed.

In more "modern" treatment, a few hundred years ago, mental patients were chained to the walls and sometimes beaten or tortured--to drive the devils out, or for the amusement of onlookers. Then, a couple of hundred years ago, they were chained to their beds. And then (as time went by) they were simply locked up. In those lockups, in addition to the mentally ill (in the present use of the words), were those who had lost their minds from syphilis, alcoholism, strokes and pellagra. To those were added people affected by too much thyroid output, as well as epileptics and those with brain infections and brain tumors. There was no attempt at treatment--what, after all, could be done?

By about 1830, such people were recognized as being ill, and France and England led the way in giving humane treatment. Some hoped that kindness would effect a cure, but it didn't help[1].

Through the years, many things were tried to cure mental illness. These included sleeping pills (since discarded), electrical shock treatment (still in use, in a very-changed form), insulin shock treatment (since discarded), lobotomy (which often removed good judgement and social sense--this procedure has been discarded), water baths and massage (since discarded), hypnosis (not much help), sodium pentothal (some psychoanalysts thought they'd bring out the truth that way--since discarded), and verbal (talking) therapy (still in use, but probably of little help for serious problems, unless drugs are also used).

Early in the twentieth century, until the use of modern drugs, about half of all hospital beds were occupied by the mentally ill. These were about one-third schizophrenics, one-third depressives, and one-third alcoholics. As of 1975, the much smaller mental wards contained 27% schizophrenics, 25% depressives, 19% alcoholics, and 29% others.[2] Thyroid-controlling drugs had enabled those with over-active thyroids to go home, and niacin (and good food) had all but eliminated pellagra, then a common cause of mental illness among the poor.

Also in the early 1900s, psychoanalysis was begun--primarily in the United States. It seemed to help those suffering from neurosis (those who were neurotic).[3] Because it often required several visits a week for several years, it could be very expensive. With the success of drug treatments, psychoanalysis has all but disappeared from the scene, with psychiatrists now rarely using verbal treatment without an accompanying drug treatment.

A breakthrough in the treatment of **schizophrenia and related illnesses** came in the late 1940s, when a French surgeon named Henri Laborit asked the Rhone-Poulenc Laboratories to make a drug with antihistamine qualities to be given before surgery. He felt that such a drug would calm his patients and thereby reduce surgical shock.

Paul Charpentier, one of the chemists at Rhone-Poulenc, started with a phenothiazine (a product of the German dye industry) and fashioned Chlorpromazine (Thorazine), in 1950. The doctor used it and noticed that it made his patients indifferent, even to serious surgery. The doctor convinced psychiatrists in Paris to try it on mental patients and it worked so well that, in just four years (in 1954), Chlorpromazine was approved for the treatment of schizophrenia in the United States. The rapid approval was due to the fact that, not only was chlorpromazine very effective, but there just weren't any other effective drugs available.

In 1953, reserpine (as alkaloid, made from the plant Rauwolfia serpentia, first used in our country as a treatment for high blood pressure) was tried and found to be effective, and joined chlorpromazine in the battle. Reserpine had been in use in India (for various purposes) for hundreds of years[4], but communications between India and the West had been very poor.

Soon after chlorpromazine and reserpine use was started, restraints in mental hospitals became rarities[5]. It's interesting that the phenothiazines were never adopted by drug addicts, as only a small percentage of what the psychotic patient takes puts them soundly to sleep.

Although neither reserpine nor the phenothiazines are tranquilizers, they were called the Major Tranquilizers[6]. One of the biggest advantages of the major tranquilizers was that they calmed psychotic patients without making them disoriented, sleepy or confused[7]. These drugs didn't correct the causes of schizophrenia, or of the various psychoses, but they did wonders at treating the symptoms and in getting people out of hospitals and into their own homes.

The success of chlorpromazine caused the pharmaceutical industry, in the next few years, to come out with several effective variations on chlorpromazine, as well as newer drugs--including haloperidol, usually called haldol, which is much in use, today. Reserpine, because of undesirable side effects and because it was considered less effective than the other medications available, fell from favor by the early 1960s.[8]

Psychoactive drugs for schizophrenia were called neuroleptics, which referred to their potential side effects. Although the early psychoactive drugs have gradually been replaced by more effective drugs with fewer side effects, it's still true that completely harmless drugs are yet to be found. While there can be side effects to the modern versions of the earlier drugs, serious side effects are extremely rare.

Side effects are best discussed with a doctor, and I won't go into them here. It's sufficient to say that, because of possible side effects, the minimal amount of medication is prescribed that (on observation) produces the desired effects. There are some modern drugs which, while quite effective, can have serious side effects and therefore require regular blood tests. In this case, it's wise that instructions be followed carefully.

Unfortunately, the earliest drugs used for schizophrenia did have more side effects than present drugs and the amounts a doctor should prescribe were unknown. As a result, doctors (in their enthusiasm, finally having an effective tool) did sometimes prescribe too much.

The result was an excess of side effects, and both

the general public and the doctors themselves were turned off, making them lean toward psychoanalysis. They felt that, while the psychoanalysts might not be effecting many obvious cures, they weren't hurting any-one, either. This wasn't quite true, considering that depressives untreated with medications were killing themselves by the thousands[9] (untreated depressives continue to do so--as well as some who are treated, but haven't been reached by the medication). This was particularly true of people with bipolar (manic depressive) illness, who were (and are) particularly vulnerable to suicide. They had to wait for lithium.

In this country, research on psychoactive drugs was stopped for a while, in the 1960s, because many influential psychiatrists still believed that mental problems were caused by family relationships. Fortunately, research in other countries continued. As late as the early 1970s, in this country, psychiatrists were still arguing about whether mental illness was caused by psychology or biology. Today, most doctors agree that biology is far-and-away the primary cause of mental problems, and the average psychiatrist spends most of his time deciding which medications to use, keeping an ongoing observation of their effects and making adjustments to them.

Most of the modern drugs were produced by chemists who took earlier successful drugs and added or subtracted a little, here and there, to or from the molecule. The resulting substances were then tried. When one of these drugs produced superior results, it (too) was taken to the lab and more additions and subtractions were tried.

In the mid-1960s, long-acting drugs in slow-release preparations, given by injections, were introduced for the treatment of schizophrenia[10]. Haldol is often given in this manner. Besides making for an even and gradual dispensing of the medication, it bypasses a tendency on the part of some to forget to take their medications and a tendency on the part of others to throw their medications away.

In addition to drugs for the treatment of schizophrenia, the 1950s brought out the **antidepressive drugs** called the **tricyclics**, which have a moderate **serotonin reuptake inhibition**--that is to say, they have the ability to decrease the removal of the transmitter serotonin from the synapse, thereby allowing a buildup of serotonin in the synapse. They were evolved from a substance called iminodibenzyl, first described in 1889[11]. In 1948, over forty compounds were synthesized from it, and among these compounds was found imipramine (Tofranil), which came on the market in 1957[12]. It was first tried as a treatment for psychosis (schizophrenia, etc.) and found ineffective--but, in 1958, it was found to be very effective against depression[13].

From imipramine were synthesized several other drugs, all of which were active against depression. Tofranil (imipramine) is still one of the tricyclics marketed in the United States for the treatment of depressive and related illnesses. There's also at least one tetracyclic. (As in a child's tricycle, the name refers to the number of "wheels" in the molecule.)

The tricyclics are very effective against depression but, like most of the medications used in mental illness, are less narrow in their effect than might be desired. One problem seems to be the decrease of a transmitter called acetylcholine, bringing about a higher pulse rate, more rapid breathing and other effects--which things are undesirable on a permanent basis, particularly in the elderly. Another problem involves the hormone histamine.

One drug which had its start in the early 1950s (as a treatment for tuberculosis) was Iproniazid. By 1957, it had been superseded as an antitubercular by other drugs which were more effective for that purpose. But, in the meantime, it was found to be a very effective antidepressant (it may have been the first **monoamine oxidase inhibitor--MAOI**). (After serotonin is released into the synapse it's taken back up for reuse, or for destruction by monoamine oxidase--MAO. The monoamine oxidase inhibitors--MAOIs--inhibit this destruction.) Unfortunately, Iproniazid was found to have some toxicity to the liver and a few cases of jaundice developed, so it had to be withdrawn from the market at that time. I understand that it may now be used in medication-resistant cases of depression or panic disorder (with close observation of the liver).

The monoamine oxidase inhibitors now in use are close relatives of Iproniazid. There was a time when these later MAOIs were thought to be dangerous, too, but it was found that the user of the drug had only to stay away from certain foods[14]. This is all well and good, but the problem arises that, when dealing with patients who may be suicidal, even that bit of information can be dangerous. So, the prescribing doctor has to know the patient.

The treatments for the four principal groups of **depressive** illness--**major, psychotic, atypical** and **bipolar**--are somewhat different from each other.

The treatment of **MAJOR DEPRESSION** is usually started with the tricyclics. Prozac or another SSRI can be tried (the SSRIs--Selective Serotonin Reuptake Inhibitors--are discussed below), and the last but most effective treatment is electroconvulsant (electric shock) therapy.

The treatment of **PSYCHOTIC DEPRESSION** is usually started with a combination of a tricyclic and an antipsychotic drug, with the possibility of electroconvulsant therapy (which is very effective).

ATYPICAL DEPRESSION is usually started with either a monoamine oxidase inhibitor (MAOI) or an SSRI such as Prozac. Since, with the MAOIs, watching what you eat is very important, Prozac may now be the treatment of choice for this problem.

BIPOLAR AFFECTIVE DISORDER (manic-depressive illness) never responded satisfactorily to the earlier medications for either depressive or psychotic illness. Not until lithium carbonate was tried was considerable success found.

Prozac is a successful drug which was evolved from an antihistamine. The search for Prozac began at

Eli Lilly in the 1960s. Several workers with converging skills conceived, synthesized and tested many compounds. Having observed other successful drugs, they were trying to find one which was <u>specifically</u> active in the conservation of <u>serotonin</u> at synapses, and which therefore didn't produce undesired side effects by interfering with other transmitters. In 1971, Solomon Snyder of Johns Hopkins University visited Eli Lilly and gave a talk which supplied them with one of their final methods for searching. In June of 1974, they published a report on the use of a substance (fluoxetine--later named Prozac) on rat brain--but it took another thirteen years, until December of 1987, before Prozac was approved for humans[15].

Prozac had some trouble gaining government approval, as it was compared to the tricyclics against major depression and is only as effective as the tricyclics, against this problem (and has to be superior, I believe, to gain approval). One thing which worked in Prozac's favor, however, was that there were very few side effects--which carries with it an additional benefit: the patient is much less likely to discontinue the medication.

Prozac was found especially effective for atypical depression, depression with anxiety, and OCD (obsessive compulsive disorder)--and may eventually be used as a complete replacement for the MAOIs. Prozac has been found relatively safe on those occasions when it has been taken in suicidal overdose and, in normal doses, patients report not feeling the effects of the drug, as they did when on MAOIs or tricyclics[16].

Several other drugs similar to Prozac have come on the market in the last few years. They are also very effective and have the same almost-total lack of side effects. They, too, are intended to conserve serotonin in the synapse or to improve the reception of serotonin on the downstream side of the synapse, and are all called (along with Prozac) **selective serotonin reuptake inhibitors** (SSRIs). (When Prozac is mentioned as a medication, in this book, it usually means Prozac or another selective serotonin reuptake inhibitor). One precaution which must be taken with Prozac and the other SSRIs is to not take them in conjunction with an MAOI[17].

The history of lithium is interesting. Lithium was discovered, as an element, in 1817. Throughout the 1800s, it was tried as a cure for many problems and, about the time of the Civil War, was tried as a cure for various types of mental derangement. An American, Dr. John Aulde, and a Dane, Dr. Carl Lange, called the world's attention to its use as an antidepressant in the mid-1880s[18].

Lithium salts were tried as a salt substitute in the 1940s, which resulted in toxicity problems and a fall from favor in medical circles. However, it wasn't much later that J.F.J. Cade (in the 1940s) and M. Schou (in the early 1950s) showed it to be effective in the treatment of bipolar depression[19].

Treatment with lithium is usually started with an accompanying antidepressive drug if the patient is in the depressed part of the cycle, with an antipsychotic if in the manic phase, and is given alone if in the intermediate normal phase. The other drugs are then usually discontinued as that phase disappears. Lithium is effective against both the manic and the depressive phases of bipolar illness[20].

There are precautionary lab tests to take, before starting on lithium, but that's best discussed with your doctor. Lithium isn't usually recommended for the elderly or during pregnancy, and is only effective on about 80% of others. Although they aren't as effective as lithium, when it works, there is a choice of several other drugs which can be taken by those twenty percent of people on whom lithium doesn't work, and by those for whom it isn't recommended.

GENERALIZED ANXIETY DISORDER (GAD) is oftentimes treated with the benzodiazepines, like Librium or Valium, or with a drug like buspirone (BuSpar).

PANIC DISORDER is often treated with the antidepressive tricyclics, with MAOIs, or with Prozac. Benzodiazepines are sometimes used.

PHOBIAS can be treated with MAOIs, or with beta blockers, and are sometimes treated with Prozac. (Beta blockers don't cure the phobias, but do slow the heart rate and lower the blood pressure. This makes phobias easier to bear, and easier to conceal from others.)[21]

OBSESSIVE COMPULSIVE DISORDER (OCD) is often treated with antidepressant drugs like Prozac.

BORDERLINE PERSONALITY DISORDER

has been difficult to treat. At the moment, Prozac and the other serotonin reuptake inhibitors seem to be the medications of choice. Tricyclic drugs don't seem to be effective on it. MAOIs have been found somewhat effective, but the impulsive nature of these patients makes it hard to keep them on a restricted diet. Lithium has been of some help, as have temporal lobe epilepsy drugs. Low doses of antipsychotics are still in the experimental stage.

Now, I'll add a few words about **electrical shock treatment** (electroconvulsive therapy--ECT).

When electrical shock treatments were first used, the amount and kind of electrical power needed was uncertain, the patient was awake during the treatment and extremely uncomfortable and, when the shock was given, the patient's arms and legs flew about so violently that broken bones were not unusual. Moreover, since it wasn't known who would be helped by the procedure, it was overused--as judged by present knowledge. In addition, it may also have been used repeatedly on people who obviously weren't being helped.

Now, however, the types of problems that can be helped are known, the amount and kind of current to be used are known and closely controlled, the patient is under anesthesia and knows and remembers nothing of the procedure and a shot is given to prevent the limbs from flying about (the only twitching is said to be in the toes).

ECT is used primarily for the treatment of major

depression, but it is sometimes used for patients with bipolar depression who are unresponsive to medications, and for other problems. It isn't usually effective in treating atypical depression, but is particularly effective in treating psychotic depression. (As of 1985, ECT was used almost exclusively for severe depression.)[22]

Although no one knows why electrical shock treatments work, they are reported to work extremely well, as noted above. Nevertheless, shock treatments are usually used only when medications are unsuccessful in treating severe depression, or if the patient is quite suicidal, or pregnant (when drugs might harm the fetus), or is quite old, or has other medical problems where medications might be dangerous.

Shock treatments are usually restricted to the above cases, not because of problems in the treatment, but because of public antipathy to the procedure, resulting from the early use (and the movie "One Flew Over The Cuckoo's Nest"). Electrical shock treatment is, despite public feelings, still the most successful procedure now in use for major depression and has a very high cure rate, even when drugs have been ineffective. (As of 1985, more than 100,000 patients a year were receiving ECT.)[23]

That said, I hope that when and if my suggestions are used, these treatments will become a thing of the past. One can even hope that the tricyclics, MAOIs and even Prozac (and the other serotonin reuptake inhibitors) will also be unneeded.

Ch 6

HOW MENTAL ILLNESS ATTACKED
MY FAMILY AND HOW I FOUGHT BACK

This chapter was originally part of an unpublished novel I wrote quite a few years ago, with the idea of getting this information published. I spent a lot of years working on the novel, and it was said to be OK--but it was felt, by those in a position to know, that it had too many non-fiction chapters to be publishable as a novel. This chapter tells how the present book came to be written, tells some of the conjectures I've made on mental illness in the last thirty-some years (some of which later chapters may make unimportant), and gives the beginnings of what I now offer. Let's hear what that old chapter had to say:

How did I become involved in the problems of the mentally-ill? Our eldest son, (now 46), has severe mental problems and has to take a very heavy load of medications. But he still manages to be pleasant, still urges us

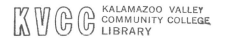

to bring him things so that he can put them in a collection for the poor, and gives ten to twenty percent of his tiny income to the Salvation Army and similar organizations. He managed to irritate his mother, recently, by giving away a jacket we'd given him. He felt that he shouldn't have two jackets, when another fellow didn't have any.

As a boy, he was fun-loving and very bright. One would have thought he was heading toward a very happy and successful life.

I remember clearly the evening we learned we were in trouble. My wife had just put the kids to bed. She came into the living room and said she was worried about something our son had told her (he was then eight).

It turned out that he wasn't able to control his thoughts. I offered as much comfort as I could, but we took him to a psychiatrist as soon as possible and the worst was confirmed. It turned out that the problem had started at the age of seven. A voice had sworn at him, claiming to be God and saying that he was no damned good. He said he knew it wasn't God, because God wouldn't talk like that.

After getting our son started with professional help, I began reading about mental illness. It didn't take long to become convinced that mental problems are caused by improper body chemistry.

But during the talks my wife and I had with the psychiatrists, who (even then) helped people with medications (which had to work thru chemistry), the doctors made it clear that they had no intention of discussing body chemistry with me. They said that, since I was talking about chemistry, I must be trying to avoid taking my proper blame. They believed that mental illness in children was caused by "bad parenting."

I wondered, at the time, how many innocent parents were suffering at the hands of psychiatrists and psychologists because of that theory--in addition to the heavy load they were already carrying, with their mentally-ill children.

It was a serious blow to me to learn that the psychiatrists, as well-intentioned as they were, didn't have the slightest idea what was causing our son's problems. Fortunately, there were quite a few books, written by biological chemists, which gave the results of many blood tests, urine tests, etc., and made attempts to account for the results. Reading these books, I felt I could come to understand these things and possibly help our son.

Fortunately, those working in the psychiatric field are at least as smart as the rest of us. They finally accepted the idea that since mental problems could be improved through chemistry, and since severe problems could be caused by taking drugs like LSD, mental problems probably were a result of body chemistry.

With the idea of becoming a doctor and helping our son, I went back to college. But my job took me out of town too often for me to be able to learn as much as those who were there every day--and my grades weren't going to get me into medical school. Nor was I being much of a husband or a father--out of town half the time and at school the other half. So, after a year, I think I was right in dropping out. Oh, maybe I was wrong--it left me without any educational "qualifications."

Since then, although I don't have any certificates on the wall or much advanced education, figuring out the causes of mental illness has been a big part of my life. Until our son became ill, I almost never opened a book. Since then, I've read several hours a day--mostly on science subjects.

To find a cure for mental illness, all by myself, may have been too much to expect. But the trouble was that, though lots of work and money went into the housing of the mentally-ill (by many levels of government and both inside and outside of hospitals), and lots of money went to psychiatrists and psychologists, I felt that our federal government wasn't spending nearly enough on research. At the rate things were going, a cure would take another fifty years. (nearly forty years have gone by)

So, I read and kept my eyes open for possible causes of the unpleasant experiences that those with mental illness were having. I wasn't looking for psychological discussions, like those used by psychiatric workers in their everyday talks with patients. They have an impossible job--trying to lead people in dreamland (more or less) toward reality. (At the same time, they do decide just what their patient's problems are, what medications to give them, what changes to make in those medications to make their patient's lives more endurable--and most important, they may help prevent their suicides.)

I set out looking for physical, chemical, correctible causes of mental problems--something most psychiatrists weren't qualified to do. But if they weren't qualified, I was almost infinitely less qualified! To say the least, mental problems are hard to work on from a position of ignorance. But I remembered the elder Henry Ford's system of switching foremen from place to place, as they didn't know what was impossible and they did it anyway.

I finally realized that even the experts in chemical laboratories not only didn't know what caused mental illness--they didn't even agree, between themselves, on possible causes.

In time, I did form some opinions of my own. I accepted one old theory that some mental problems may be symptoms of an incomplete transfer from sleep to wakefulness. But even if that were so, I didn't know what could cause it.

Early on, I realized that mental illness might be caused by bacteria or viruses reaching the brain and setting up comfortable homes. But I felt that that had probably been thoroughly checked in autopsies on those who had been mentally ill. In any event, the psychiatrists told me that they felt that such germs would be more likely to cause severe physical illness.

Among the things I learned, in my studies, was that many of those who suffer from mental illness have a low bloodsugar level. They also frequently have a shortage of a substance called tryptophan (an amino acid--a protein building block) in their blood. A lot of blood goes to the brain to supply its needs and, in addition to oxygen, two of its greatest needs seem to be enough sugar (in the form of glucose) and enough tryptophan. I was sure that the brain needed all of the amino acids, but came to believe that the reported shortage of tryptophan in the blood of many of the mentally-ill was critically important.

The psychiatrists told me that a low bloodsugar level wasn't important unless it caused unconsiousness. But, in spite of what they said, I thought sugar was important too, because sugar is the primary energy source the cells we think with use--possibly the only energy source they use.

I was surprised to read that the shortage of tryptophan in the blood of the mentally-ill continued-- even when large amounts of tryptophan were added to their diets (this is said not to be so, in those not mentally-ill)! And taking tryptophan supplements, which some health food stores were selling in recent years, was even found to cause some serious problems. (I later learned that they were very serious problems. About five thousand users became ill and thirty-eight died of a bone marrow disease, which was said to be linked to an impurity in a specific shipment from Japan. U.S. Health authorities have never completely accepted that theory, and were still leery of tryptophan supplements, the last I heard.)

I read that mental patients, besides their tendency to low bloodsugar and the shortage of tryptophan in their blood, oftentimes also have an excess of something called indole in their intestinal waste. Scientists had lots of theories about the tryptophan and the indole. They'd even found brain chemistry which used tryptophan and produced some indole.

But although they were trying, I thought they were still on the wrong track. At least, I thought I knew where the tryptophan was going and where the indole was coming from--and it was a lot simpler than brain chemistry.

I supposed that some people's intestines might be unable to transfer enough tryptophan to the blood. But I'd read about what seemed a more probable answer, in a book on bacteriology. The book said that the main bacterium of the intestines--an E. *coli* relative of the one that causes food poisoning--when grown in a dish and deprived of the sugars it normally "eats," can switch to an alternate food--tryptophan. And one waste product of that switch is--indole[1]. (Another is a substance called skatole.)

(Some may argue that, since most amino acids are removed at the small intestine, the E. *coli* bacteria of the large intestine can't affect the tryptophan level. But, since the indole and skatole levels in the intestinal wastes are much higher in those with pellagra and schizophrenia, and since these are waste products of E. *coli* consumption of tryptophan in the large intestine, tryptophan apparently does pass to the large intestine.)

I assumed that some of the E. *coli* bacteria consume tryptophan in everyone's intestines, because the indole and skatole are largely responsible for the characteristic odor of the feces--bathroom odor, one might delicately put it.

Anyway, I decided that the mentally-ill folks, who have the shortage of tryptophan in their blood, may have that shortage because they have a variety of the *E. coli* bacteria in their intestines which especially enjoys eating tryptophan. Or maybe those folks have some chemical difference from other people which causes their ordinary *E. coli* to switch diets--from a lot of sugar and a little tryptophan, to a little sugar and a lot of tryptophan. And maybe, when they're given extra tryptophan in their food, they don't get any more into their blood because their intestinal bacteria are having a feast--tryptophan for the appetizer, tryptophan for the main course and tryptophan for dessert.

And maybe those bacterial waste products, like the indole and skatole, cause the problems people have with the tryptophan supplements.

The bacteriology book said that when sugars were withheld from the *E. coli* in a laboratory dish, and the bacteria did their switch to eating tryptophan, the shift could be stopped by adding a substance called pyruvic acid--which, as the book pointed out, is a normal body substance[2]. (Pyruvic acid is produced in cells by glycolysis, in the initial breakdown of glucose to obtain usable energy in the form of ATP.)

Aha! I'd thought. Why not assume that, in some people with mental problems, those bacteria have shifted more completely to eating tryptophan--and why not try to get some of that pyruvic acid stuff into those people's intestines to try to stop the shift?

I remember going out and buying that bottle of the pretty red pyruvic acid, and taking it to the medical research company over by the university. I guess I looked pretty simple when I asked what it would cost me to have capsules filled with the stuff and tried out on laboratory animals.

The pleasant oriental gentleman, who received me, politely informed me that "it's awfully hard to convince rats that they should swallow capsules--and it would take a very special capsule not to dissolve until past the stomach--and even if my people were able to accomplish the feat manually, with that special capsule, satisfying government requirements in testing your idea would cost more that a million dollars."

That was a long time ago, and I suspect that those very special capsules are very common, now--my blood pressure pills may come in them.

But that didn't help my problem, then. So, I had to thank the fellow and find my way out. But I didn't give up. All I'd read had made me agree (with the writers of several books) that at least some forms of mental illness are linked to the lack of tryptophan in the blood. And I thought I was right about that shortage being caused by the bacteria of the intestines eating the stuff.

I sat in the car, that day, and pondered the problem. I thought about trying to find those very special capsules and taking the pyruvic acid, myself--to see if it was safe--but if it ruined my health, where would my wife and kids be?

So I thought, as I drove home, I'll just have to start over again. Let's see--if mentally-ill people have a variety of *E. coli* that prefers tryptophan, that's for a lab to check--it's beyond my capability. But if normal bacteria are switching to eating tryptophan because of some difference in the ill person's body chemistry, or whatever, maybe I can figure out what that difference is.

How the hell am I going to do that! I asked myself. I'm not a chemist or a bacteriologist or a biologist! I don't know anything about those subjects, compared to what one needs to know, to do that sort of thing!

A possible (but looking back, perhaps a far-out) clue to the answer came when I read about a hormone called **glucagon**. Glucagon, it seemed, was one of a pair of hormones (the other was **insulin**) which together had the job of regulating the level of sugar in the blood. While **insulin's job** was to keep the bloodsugar level from being too high, by encouraging body cells to consume more sugar and the liver to convert and store glucose as a substance called glycogen (it's also stored in the muscles), **glucagon's job** was to keep the bloodsugar level high enough by causing the conversion of glycogen back to glucose.

I came up with the tentative theory that glucagon might also cause cells to consume less sugar, and that intestinal bacteria might be switching foods because some glucagon was getting into the intestines and stopping the bacteria from eating sugar--making them do their switch to tryptophan.

Glucagon is made in several places in the body, including the walls of the intestines. Most of it seems to be made in the pancreas, from which it passes into the blood. But I read in a comparative anatomy text that the pancreas may have as many as three ducts to the intestine, and maybe one of those ducts is usable by glucagon and enters the intestine downstream of a lot of acid and digestive enzymes.

In the unlikely event that this (early) theory (and frankly, rather imaginative series of events) should actually be right, the harmful glucagon in the intestine may very likely be alterable with medication. But the simplest solution to the bacteria consuming the tryptophan, I'd thought, if that's what's going on, might be to find (and one can now add, "or genetically produce") a variety of intestinal *E. coli* bacterium which can't consume tryptophan, or can consume very little of it (and I'll now add, "but can still produce vitamin K, and any other needed vitamins it now produces"), and then to do a switch--one person at a time. One thing that bothered me about this solution was the possibility that the original bacteria might take over again, after the switch. On the other hand, if the new bacteria are able to hold their own and multiply, in the presence of the bacteria already in the intestine, just getting a tiny culture of the new bacteria to the intestine may do the job.

I read an article in Scientific American[3] (in 1989) that convinced me that I was on the right track. The article said that people with serious depression problems sometimes feel less depressed after eating carbohydrates-- things like cupcakes and other sweets. The writers felt that this happens because of an interesting series of events: 1)the body turns the carbohydrates into sugar and this causes the pancreas to produce extra insulin; 2)the extra insulin, besides reducing the sugar level, causes body cells to remove amino acids from the blood-- **except for tryptophan**; and 3)the tryptophan (left behind, in the blood) then has less competition in getting to the brain (across the blood-brain barrier), gets there and (among other things) is made into an important substance called serotonin. The serotonin then does its normal jobs, including making those folks feel less depressed, for a while.

But one can't eat sweets and pasta all day long. And since many mentally-ill people have a lower blood-sugar level than most, their insulin production may be lower, even when they do eat sweets.

Bloodsugar and insulin relationships are too complex for me, but regardless of sugar level, the shortage of tryptophan in the blood of the mentally-ill must mean that what little tryptophan they have has lots of competition at the blood-brain barrier. Their brains, then, must get very little tryptophan and (therefore) have very little serotonin.

There isn't any doubt, anymore, that most

depressive illness is related to a lack of serotonin (most of the modern medications for depression act by decreasing the removal of serotonin from the synaptic spaces, or by decreasing the normal destruction of serotonin after it's removed), but when I read that serotonin is also involved in the control of sleeping and waking--and that LSD blocks the operation of serotonin--I decided that I had a key to one way the lack of serotonin may be involved in causing schizophrenia. Maybe the shortage of tryptophan in the blood of mental patients, by reducing the amount of serotonin in neurons, produces the same result a small amount of LSD produces--leaving those folks somewhere between being awake and asleep, as the old theory suggested, so long ago.

More recent reading makes me think that the lack of serotonin could also aggravate schizophrenia by (as strange as it sounds) reducing that portion of sleep which contains most of our dreams (called REM sleep). (Whether or not this is so, what I now feel are the causes of the depressive illnesses and schizophrenia are discussed in chapter eight, as well as probable cures for depressive illness and preventions for schizophrenia.)

At that early time, I wondered what would happen if a test group of mentally-ill people were given continuous IVs (intravenous feedings) of tryptophan, of the amounts necessary to bring their blood tryptophan levels up to that of the average person. Would some of them be "much improved," after a few weeks? (I now believe that, in the case of depression, the recovery would be dramatic--and that, though the acute schizophrenic would be helped, the chronic schizophrenic would not--except for those symptoms which may be caused by a lack of serotonin in some neurons. I do have other suggestions for helping the chronic schizophrenic, however, also covered in chapter eight.) If the tryptophan IVs were success-ful, and on the unfortunate chance that pyruvic acid were tried and found ineffective, I wondered if tryp-tophan could be injected as a slow-release medication, or by a portable unit such as is used for insulin.

I further wondered, at that time, how many of us who are considered mentally healthy have failed to be all we might have been, because of a moderate shortage of tryptophan in our blood, caused by those most-common-and-accepted bacteria in the world--the ordinary bacteria of our own intestines.

Maybe, if a worldwide switching of bacteria is eventually done, or if pyruvic acid capsules (or some other kind of capsules) are found to be successful in decreasing the bacterial consumption of tryptophan, peace and peacefulness will settle upon the whole earth.

(end of recently revised chapter from my old book)

Ch 7

Serotonin

I believe that a shortage of serotonin is the cause of and also the key to the cure of depressive mental illness.

Serotonin is a transmitter used by only a small percentage of neurons, but these neurons are critically important to our well-being. As mentioned in the previous chapter, almost all of the medications which are used to treat depressive and related illnesses work by having an effect on the serotonin usage of these neurons.

The neurons which use serotonin as a transmitter are located in the older part of the brain--the brain stem (serotonin is also used by the Pineal Body of the brain, but not as a transmitter). The brain stem is called "older" because the "lesser" animals--even the reptiles--have this much brain (and a little of what can be called cortex), and on close

examination the brains of reptiles are found to be distur-
bingly similar to our brain stem.

Most of the neurons of our brain stem which use
serotonin as a transmitter are located in the **Raphe
Nuclei**--at least, their cell bodies are--and these make up
several good-sized groups of cells (almost all the neurons
of the raphe nuclei use serotonin). The two raphe nuclei
which far and away have the most to do with the
operation of the brain are the **Dorsal** (toward the back)
Raphe and the **Medial** (in the middle) **Raphe**. (The other
raphe nuclei, which send some axons upward but go mostly to the
spinal cord, can be important too, because they--among other things
--can inhibit pain messages from the body, so that, once you've
received the pain information, the amount of pain decreases. This is
very useful, with long-term pain.)

Considering their great importance in mental
illness, there are relatively few of these serotonin-using
neurons. The Dorsal Raphe Nucleus, which puts out the
greatest number of serotonin-using axons to the rest of
the brain, is estimated to have only about 165,000
neurons[1] (out of about a hundred billion neurons in the
entire brain, you'll remember).

Although the cell bodies of most of these neurons
are in the raphe nuclei, their axons extend out to all
parts of the brain. I realize that the names of the
principal places these nuclei send their messages to may
not mean a thing to many of you: the hippocampus, the
cerebral cortex, the septal nuclei, the caudate putamen,
the hypothalamus, the thalamus and others. But to the
expert, those names ring like the names of the great cities
of the world. The serotonin-using connections to these
important areas have one thing in common--they all

depend on a sufficient supply of the amino acid tryptophan to make that serotonin.

So a shortage of tryptophan in the blood is a serious problem, because of the serotonin and other important things made from it. Each neuron of the brain that uses serotonin as a transmitter receives that tryptophan from the blood of the brain, sends it along those miniscule tubes in its tiny root-like axon to each of its individual output synapses, and each output synapse manufactures its own serotonin.

Predictably, it's not quite that simple. In addition to sending tryptophan (in vesicles) on the tubes to the synapses, the cell body manufactures (from recipes in the genetic code) both **enzymes** and **neuropeptides** and sends them to the synapses, too.

The **enzymes** speed up chemical reactions, which wouldn't go fast enough without them, at body temperature. Two different enzymes are needed in the synapses to change tryptophan to serotonin.

The **neuropeptides** are short strings of amino acids (anywhere from two to 40+ amino acids in length), which have jobs of their own to accomplish. Oftentimes, when a transmitter is released into a synapse, one or more of these neuropeptides are also released. They may coordinate in the work of the transmitter; they may influence other cells altogether (other than the ones on which the transmitting and receiving synapses are found); and they may have other jobs, about which little (so far) is known.

The serotonin-using cells have primarily an inhibiting (calming) influence on systems they go to and tend to soothe such things as one's mood and one's rising temper, as well as being involved in such diverse things as perception (understanding), and eating problems.

A shortage of serotonin in neurons extending to the frontal cortex (behind the forehead) can cause aggressive behavior toward oneself and toward others, as well as serious impulsiveness, and can result in violent acts of self-destruction. (A shortage of serotonin in the amygdala and hypothalamus may also be involved.) A shortage of serotonin in the frontal cortex (behind the forehead) has been found after criminal acts of aggression, too. The level of serotonin has been found to be particularly low in arsonists, for some reason. (It's also been noted that bodybuilding steroids may reduce serotonin levels enough to produce violence. Perhaps that has something to do with some of the violence one sees in professional sports.)

The serious depletion of serotonin in suicidally depressive people can be verified by a spinal tap. Researchers find a low level of the serotonin breakdown product 5-HIAA (otherwise known as 5-hydroxyindoleacetic acid), which finds its way from neurons to the fluid chambers of the brain (the **ventricles**), and thence to the fluid passages in and around the spinal cord, finally getting to where the tap is done. This is the way the above mentioned serotonin level of arsonists was determined. (Medications for depression, particularly the SSRIs, help one to avoid suicide not by increasing the amount of serotonin being manufactured in the synapses, but primarily by conserving the serotonin already present.)

Besides depressive illness, a host of other illnesses are alleviated by the SSRIs and other antidepressive medications. These problems include Obsessive Compulsive Disorder (OCD), Panic Disorder, eating problems, alcoholism, obesity and sleep problems. It's probable that anger, hostility, impulsivity, aggression and migraine headaches will also be found to be helped by the SSRIs. (Actually, there may be as many as fifty medical problems in which a lack of serotonin is involved, and which would probably be alleviated by an increase in serotonin.)

Alcoholism is helped, but not cured, by the SSRIs[2]. Exactly why they should help is unknown, but studies have shown a close relationship between low cerebrospinal 5-HIAA, hypoglycemia (low bloodsugar) and alcoholism.

One theory of Bipolar Affective Disorder (manic-depressive illness) is that while one's serotonin supply is too meagre in both the manic and the depressive phases of the illness, the differences between the manic and the depressive phases are brought about by a high (with the manic phase) and a low (with the depressive phase) concentration of a transmitter called norepinephrine (noradrenaline). The question remains: without the low level of serotonin, would the illness occur at all?

SEROTONIN RECEPTORS (receivers)

The more receptors are studied, the more complex they're found to be--the subject is tremendously complex. But, for our purposes, I'd like to compare the subject to the making of an automobile. There's a great amount of knowledge involved in the design, manufacture and maintenance of automobiles. Certainly such knowledge has improved automobiles in the last fifty years. But it isn't necessary to have much technical knowledge to drive a car where you want to go. The same thing applies to operating computers. And the same may hold for the brain and its receptors, as far as the cure of mental illness is concerned. If we can help to bring about cures for mental illnesses by the use of superficial peripheral knowledge, that will be good enough for me. So, let's try to get a little superficial knowledge of receptors.

All of the serotonin-using neurons of the brain need serotonin receptors (receivers) in the downstream cells (downstream in the direction of signal-flow). There are many slightly different (and a few considerably different) kinds of serotonin receptors--there may be as many as a dozen different kinds.

Part of this number is accounted for by the many different jobs serotonin has been given to do and part of it may just be duplication of effort--much like the duplication found in the genetic code--a built-in insurance policy.

But let's speculate, for a moment, and see if we can imagine some ways the body may make use of the many different serotonin receptors, for the many different "jobs." Is it possible that the body, sensing different needs, makes slight changes to the serotonin--making it more likely to be accepted by some of the receptors than the others, setting those receptors more busily to work than the rest? Or is it possible that the body, sensing these differing needs, makes the various receptors for those jobs more or less attractive to the serotonin? Or is it possible that the body changes the number of the various receptors to bring about needed results?

The last suggestion seems to be the answer. At

least, the downstream cells of people with depressive illness have been found to have an increased number of serotonin receptors (trying, perhaps, to pump a dry well).

Whatever the purpose nature had in mind for the wide variety of serotonin receptors, scientists are determined to take advantage of that variety by producing medications which will activate each type of receptor individually, getting it to be more active at its own specific job. They've had a little success in that direction and are working to accomplish more.

In any event, there are many different kinds of serotonin receptors, which can bring about a variety of results. At first, I intended to list the various serotonin receptors I could find information on, where they are found and what their jobs are thought to be. But, that seemed a little beyond this book's scope. What I am going to do is say a little about a receptor called 1A (actually 5-HT_{1A}), and then list some of the things in which serotonin receptors seem to be involved.

First of all, the 1A is found on both transmitting and receiving cells. On a transmitting cell, it's often found on those tiny root-like dendrites and on the main cell body--in both cases, apparently being used in feedback circuits to tend to keep the cell from firing. In effect, these receptors have the job of decreasing the operation (for some reason) of these cooling, soothing cells. Some scientists are hoping to disable these receptors in people with depressive illness, so that these serotonin-using cells won't be shut down.

On transmitting cell synapses, 1A also acts as an **autoreceptor**, tending to cause the cells not to fire--in effect, telling the transmitter bouton that there's enough serotonin in the synaptic space already. These receptors probably don't get much action in people with depressive illness--at least they shouldn't, since the synapses are too short of serotonin. (Both MAOIs and SSRIs make 1A autoreceptors in raphe nuclei less sensitive--less likely to tell the cell that enough serotonin is present in the synapse. After long-term treatment, this increases the effects of serotonin on downstream cells.)[3]

On receiving cells (on downstream boutons), the 1As are found primarily in the hippocampal areas of the temporal lobes of the brain--next to the ears--where the serotonin receptors can cause chemical reactions using a substance called cyclic AMP (cyclic adenosine monophosphate), which acts as a cell "second messenger." Second messengers, in these downstream cells, can produce results as divergent as opening or closing ion channels (having to do with bringing about or preventing the firing of these cells), regulating cell enzymes, or altering the outputs of genes.

In addition to being concentrated in the hippocampus, which is important in short-term memory and very important in schizophrenia (because of shrinkage), and the (adjacent) entorhinal cortex (having to do with the sense of smell), the 1A is also numerous in the septal area in the center of the brain[4] and other nuclei of the limbic system, having to do with emotions.

Receptors other than the 1A are found on transmitting cell synapses, acting as a different kind of autoreceptor--taking serotonin back out of the synaptic space into the transmitter bouton. It's worth mentioning again that once back in the transmitter bouton, the serotonin is either disposed of (by monoamine oxidase--MAO) or re-packaged for reuse (they get packed into more of those little spheres, called vesicles, which carry thousands of serotonin molecules each--perhaps as many as 10,000 serotonin molecules in each vesicle).

Interestingly, when serotonin is released, it's released in increments of one (or more) vesicles--that is, in batches of perhaps 10,000 serotonin molecules at a time, or multiples thereof. To accommodate this number of serotonin transmitter molecules, the downstream cells have a multitude of serotonin receptors.

Some serotonin receptors, on downstream receiving cells, have to do with a substance called phospho-inositide, inside the downstream cells (involved with other "second messengers"). Other serotonin receptors are found throughout the brain, performing a variety of duties, mostly inhibitory--cooling and soothing in nature. Some may be involved in the secretion of cerebrospinal fluid. (If serotonin inhibits the making of cerebrospinal fluid, a shortage of serotonin might tend to explain the enlarged ventricles found with schizophrenia--they perhaps being the result of a low-level hydro-cephalus--water on the brain. The enlarged ventricles are now, however, thought to be caused by a decrease in brain mass.)

Several different kinds of serotonin receptors are found right in the raphe nuclei, where the neurons apparently do some integrating, before going out to work.

Serotonin and its receptors are vital to our well-being. They are the most-studied transmitter and receptors of the brain, at this time.

Box 1. Tryptophan.

Tryptophan is an "essential" amino acid in the diet; that is, the body can't manufacture it.

Some sources: meat, fish, poultry, milk, cheese, eggs, dried beans, soy products, seafood, etc. A mixture of foods is best, along with nuts, whole wheat products, etc.

Some products the body makes from tryptophan:

    niacin (see ch. 8)
    serotonin (ch. 5, 6, 7, 8, 9)
    melatonin (ch. 9)
    NAD   (ch. 8 and glossary)
    NADH (ch. 8 and glossary)
    NADP   (ch. 8 and glossary)
    NADPH (ch. 8 and glossary)

Ch 8

WHAT REALLY CAUSES MENTAL ILLNESS?
WHAT CAN BE DONE ABOUT IT?

As I mentioned in chapter six, what convinced me long ago that I could influence the treatment of mental illness was reading, in several books, that the blood of many of the mentally-ill was short of tryptophan. One of these books stated that the blood level of tryptophan didn't rise when these patients were fed large amounts of tryptophan or tryptophan-rich foods (as a normal person's bloodlevel is said to rise), and that the bowel waste of many of the mentally-ill had an excess of the substances indole and skatole.

When I learned that the *E. coli* bacteria of the intestine can, when there's not enough sugar present, consume tryptophan and discard indole and skatole, I felt that those bacteria had to be consuming the tryptophan.

Since, in all of us, indole and skatole produce the

normal odor of the feces, we may all suffer to some extent from this bacterial consumption. But I believe that those with serious mental problems suffer a more complete bacterial depletion of the intestinal tryptophan.

As mentioned in chapter six, pyruvic acid can cause *E. coli* bacteria, in a dish in the lab, to stop consuming tryptophan. I suggest that pyruvic acid capsules should be tested, to see if they can safely produce this desirable result in the human intestine. I also expressed my belief that a variety of *E. coli* intestinal bacterium which can't consume so much tryptophan (but can still produce vitamin K, and any other necessary vitamins now produced) can be found or genetically created--and I also urge that that be done.

When the blood of the brain has plenty of tryptophan, serotonin-using cells get enough of it to produce needed serotonin. But if the blood of the brain is short of tryptophan, those neurons get too little of it and their output synapses are short of serotonin and fail to transmit messages strongly enough, or often enough. I believe such disruptions of synaptic messages, caused by a shortage of tryptophan, to be the cause of the depressive illnesses.

When a serotonin-using neuron "fires," serotonin is put out into the synapse, delivering the cell's message. The cell then takes it back up again and either repackages it for reuse or destroys it. As has been mentioned, most of the medications used to treat depression (and a host of other problems) work by inhibiting this reuptake of serotonin, or this destruction of serotonin, or by increasing the effective use of the serotonin which reaches the synaptic space. These medications include the tricyclics, the monoamine oxidase inhibitors, Prozac and its fellow serotonin reuptake inhibitors, and even lithium. (Lithium may also cause an increase in the amount of tryptophan reaching the neurons, at least initially.)

But if these medications, which are used to treat a multitude of mental ills, all work with serotonin, we'd better take a closer look at serotonin and what it does (many people are studying it). Most importantly, we need to find out if serotonin is really in short supply in neurons in those with depressive and related illnesses, as I'm sure it is (it has been recently reported that a number of researchers say it's 20-25 percent lower in those at high risk of suicide)[1], and we need to find out if increasing (somewhat) the amount of tryptophan in the blood of the brain--thereby increasing (somewhat) the serotonin level in neurons which have been short of tryptophan--will make all of the medications for depressive illness unnecessary.

The increase of (normally produced) serotonin in neurons in which its level has been too low, and the decrease of the need for medications to raise that level, are what I am trying to accomplish in depressive illness.

There are several problems involved in doing this. One problem is that the blood-brain barrier, whose primary job is to protect the brain from harmful substances, passes amino acids to the brain according to their **relative** blood concentration. (If the amount of one amino acid in the blood increases, while the others stay the same, an increased amount of the first amino acid will pass the blood-brain barrier, to the brain. If the amount of the first one stays the same, but the others decrease, the same thing will happen.) If too little tryptophan is present, too little will be passed.

You may remember from chapter six that **when a person eats carbohydrates** (sugars and/or starches) the sugar level of the blood is raised, which causes the pancreas to put out insulin, which not only lowers the sugar level but also **raises** the **relative** level of **tryptophan** in the blood by causing body cells to **remove other amino acids** from the blood. Since, after the partial removal of these other amino acids, the level of tryptophan is **relatively higher** than it was, the blood-brain barrier passes more of it to the brain--the result being more tryptophan to the neurons, more tryptophan to the synapses, more serotonin into the synaptic spaces and (temporarily) less sufferering from depression. All this, just by consuming carbohydrates.

These findings on how insulin in the blood affects the levels of amino acids in the blood have certainly been verified.

But now I propose that, by restricting the consumption of tryptophan by intestinal bacteria (either by replacing the bacteria with a strain that can't consume as much of it, or with pyruvic acid), we cause the **intestinal** level of tryptophan to rise, thus causing the intestine to pass more of it to the blood of the body.

When the additional intestinal tryptophan has reached the blood of the body, the **relative level** of tryptophan in that blood will be higher (relative to the other amino acids)--**without changing the levels of the other amino acids.** This should increase the amount of tryptophan which passes the blood-brain barrier, increasing the amount of tryptophan to reach the neurons which have been short of tryptophan, increasing the amount of serotonin in the synapses which have needed more serotonin--**and do so without raising the insulin level, lowering the bloodsugar level or interfering** (significantly) **with the passage of other amino acids to the brain.**

It's been found that the concentration of tryptophan in the brain is the rate-limiting factor (by a factor of thirty)[2] in the production of serotonin. Raising the tryptophan level in the brain **will,** therefore, increase the level of serotonin **in neurons which need an increase.**

It has been asked how increasing the tryptophan level of the intestine by controlling intestinal bacteria differs from increasing the tryptophan level of the intestine with tryptophan additives. The answer is that I consider the problem with the additives to be either that the story of the contaminated shipment of tryptophan is true, or that the waste products of the intestinal bacteria (after consuming tryptophan) are harmful. Certainly, tryptophan is needed in the blood.

Raising the tryptophan level of the blood too much, however, would produce toxic effects in the liver[3]. That's why I consider it important to provide plenty of tryptophan to the intestine in the normal diet, **prevent bacteria from consuming it,** and then let the **body** control how much of it is passed to the blood. It's my opinion that, because of the intestinal *E. coli*, the blood level of tryptophan is somewhat lower than optimum (and thus the brain levels of tryptophan and serotonin also somewhat lower than optimum) even in the average normal person, and that that's one reason for the aggressive nature of man (as suggested by the low level of the serotonin breakdown product--5-HIAA--in the cerebrospinal fluid of people with agression problems).

I don't think that the intestine will pass a toxically-high level of tryptophan to the blood, **even if the intestinal *E. coli* are controlled or replaced,** if we just consume a well-rounded diet. The body is too well regulated for that.

So, by replacing the *E. coli* bacteria in our intestines, or by taking pyruvic acid capsules to control them, it's possible that we could eliminate or radically reduce the incidence of depressive illness. **But the cure of schizophrenia is, or may be, an entirely different problem.**

The most obvious difference between the depressive illnesses and schizophrenia is that the symptoms are much improved with the use of completely different medications--and these medications act on entirely different transmitters (most schizophrenia medications are involved with the transmitter dopamine). Still, the fact remains that, with both schizophrenia and depressive illness, there is a considerable time lag between the actions of the medications on the transmitters and the signs of symptom improvement. No one knows why. Why do the delays exist? What is actually causing these illnesses? I'm satisfied that depressive problems are caused by a chronic shortage of blood tryptophan, causing a chronic shortage of serotonin--but what about schizophrenia? I'm convinced that schizophrenia is also caused by a chronic shortage of blood tryptophan, **but for two reasons--partly because of a serotonin shortage, and partly because of an additional problem.**

First, I would like to list some bits of information that may show that a shortage of serotonin in the output synapses of the raphe neurons may be part of the problem, in schizophrenia. Please stay with me through this list of items **for the experts** (and would the experts please be patient with the short explanations, inserted here and there for others), because **after listing them I'll discuss the second way that blood tryptophan is vitally important in schizophrenia.** Here goes...

A) LSD produces a severe schizophrenia-like reaction, and;

   A1) LSD reduces the rate of firing of serotonin neurons in the raphe nucleus[4]. This seems to be brought about through feedback connections to dendritic autoreceptors[5].

B) Schizophrenia has been described as being stuck somewhere between being awake and being asleep, and;

   B1) Destroying the raphe nuclei is said to eliminate sleep in cats[6].

B2) The raphe nuclei have connections to the locus coeruleus (another brainstem nucleus), the destruction of which eliminates REM (rapid eye movement) sleep[7].

B3) It's been said that serotonin-using neurons need rest, and that they do rest during REM sleep.

B4) Sleep deprivation can produce a 20% decrease in brain serotonin[8].

B5) The raphe nuclei have connections to the reticular formation (a group of neurons in the brain stem, near the raphe nuclei), which controls the level of consciousness.

(I wonder if a shortage of serotonin in the Raphe neurons could bring about a reduced level of consciousness--to between being awake and asleep--by affecting the reticular formation.)

C) Complex interrelationships between serotonin and dopamine systems have been described.[9] (again, dopamine is the transmitter at which most medications for schizophrenia are aimed)

D) Several aberrations in platelet 5-HT[10] (serotonin in blood platelets), and CSF 5-HIAA[11] (the breakdown product of serotonin found in cerebrospinal fluid) are also found in schizophrenia.

E) Animal studies have shown that serotonin may modulate dopamine activities[12].

F) But: Several medications for schizophrenia, including clozapine, risperidone, ritanserin and setoperone have 5-HT antagonistic properties[13] (they're antagonistic to serotonin).

The above items may help the experts to see how a shortage of serotonin may cause some of the problems of schizophrenia, but I believe schizophrenia has **two** causes--the one being related to the shortage of serotonin, and the other being **a small chronic shortage of nicotinic acid** (niacin), in the blood. To supplement the niacin received in food consumed, the body (in addition to the niacin manufactured by bacteria in the intestine), makes it from **tryptophan** (with the help of pyridoxine--vitamin B6[14]. Thiamine and riboflavin--vitamins B1 and B2--are also involved[15].). A shortage of tryptophan in the blood reduces this supplementation of niacin.

All this is to say that **I believe schizophrenia is caused by a chronic low level of pellagra** (a formerly prevalent deficiency disease, caused by eating a diet short of tryptophan and niacin, whose progressive symptoms were then called the four Ds: dementia, dermatitis, diarrhea and death). This pellagra of schizophrenia is not fullblown pellagra, with all its symptoms, but a chronic low level (where the symptoms don't progress past dementia).

I believe that this low-level pellagra is brought about, not by a shortage of tryptophan in the diet (as is the case with full-blown pellagra), but--like the depressive illnesses--by the *E. coli* bacteria of the intestine consuming too much tryptophan, before it can get to the blood.

Since **full-blown** pellagra has been all but gone in our country since about 1930, few will remember that, in full-blown pellagra, mental problems such as the loss of short-term memory, decrease in useful intelligence, and symptoms of psychotic illness and depression were known to sometimes precede the physical symptoms of the pellagra by weeks or months[16].

It was said at that time that the symptoms of low-level pellagra were unknown. (I suggest that they are finally known.)

The illness called pellagra was found to be avoidable by maintaining a well-rounded diet (if one could afford it), and was later found treatable with niacin. Unfortunately, it was also learned long ago that acute (recent) mental problems caused by pellagra respond well to niacin supplements, but chronic (of long duration) cases don't--thus, if schizophrenia is partly caused by a chronic low-level of pellagra, people with chronic schizophrenia will probably still be unhelped by vitamin consumption.

I accept that, when pellagra was still common, acute mental problems caused by pellagra responded well to niacin and chronic cases didn't. I now therefore urge regular precautionary niacin supplements for the young, not in excessive amounts, to eliminate part of the cause of schizophrenia (niacin won't affect the lack of serotonin); and niacin supplement therapy for those with acute schizophrenia, with the hope of improvement or cure; and some niacin for those with chronic schizophrenia, with the hope of keeping things from getting worse.

Since both causes of schizophrenia (the lack of

serotonin and the lack of niacin) are related to a low level of tryptophan in the blood, the following questions become important: when did the tryptophan shortage start, when does low-level schizophrenia-pellagra becomes chronic, and what determines when niacin will no longer help?

I would like to ask **the experts** these questions:

1)If the bacterial decrease of tryptophan in the blood has caused a lack of supplemented niacin, thus decreasing the masses of NAD/NADH and NADP/NADPH in the body, would it be possible to supply NAD/NADH and/or NADP/NADPH to the body? (niacin being one of the starting substances in the manufacture of NAD[17]--**NAD/NADH being vital to the production of usable energy in all cells.** NADPII, derived from NAD, is important in the synthesis of fatty acids and needed cholesterol--cholesterol being one component of the myelin sheaths which insulate nerve axons. I wonder if a shortage of tryptophan, and thus of niacin, and thus of NADPH could be a factor in illnesses where myelin is involved...).

2)The inner mitochondrial membrane is reported to be impermeable to NADH[18], at least in some cells[19]. It is further reported that NAD$^+$ cannot permeate the inner membrane[20]. But, since mitochondria reproduce by division, halving the amount of NAD/NADH and other substances in the matrix of each, must not NAD and all other substances needed after reproduction either be produced from the mitochondrial genome (using niacin /nicotinamide) or pass the inner membrane? If the latter, and NAD/NADH is short when this takes place, will the mitochondrion be forever short of these substances?

3)Is it possible that the lower blood sugar level of

some of the mentally ill is caused by this shortage of NAD/NADH, by so disturbing the citric acid cycle throughout the body that the mitochondria increase glycolysis for energy production, requiring more glucose consumption?

4)Could this same disruption of energy production, in the substantia nigra, be a contributing factor in Parkinson's disease?   (end of questions for the experts)

My oldest son may be able to give us some indication as to the time required for schizophrenia to become chronic. He started to have severe problems at the age of seven. In his early twenties, fifteen years after it started, he went to California as a member of a band. He was already on considerable medication at that age, but was on and off it, so his memory may not be perfect. He claims that at that time he took niacin supplements (of megavitamin size) for three years, with no noticeable help. The problem had probably long-since been chronic, so far as niacin help was concerned.

But the problem may have become chronic soon after the symptoms of schizophrenia first appeared. It may turn out that niacin supplements will have to be taken as soon as (or even before) symptoms appear, to keep schizophrenia from becoming chronic.

The solution is that, if my suggestions are taken and the bacteria of the intestine are replaced (or pyruvic acid capsules are successfully used), increased blood tryptophan may cure acute cases of schizophrenia-pellagra; new cases may not start; plenty of serotonin will be made, doing much to help those with depressive problems (and possibly schizophrenics); and the children of the future may grow up without schizophrenia or depressive illness. And since the mitochondria of the entire body need an adequate supply of niacin, our entire bodies may benifit. (The mitochondria are small bodies in our cells which, as mentioned earlier, convert--primarily--the energy in glucose to a usable form.)

Truly, the world needs someone to go to work on the tryptophan metabolism of the intestinal *E. coli* bacterium. And, as more fully noted for the experts a few paragraphs back and here noted again **for the experts**, I believe an attempt should be made to get NAD/NADH to neuronal mitochondria, as well as NADP/NADPH to the brain, as possible ways to help those with chronic schizophrenia.

In regard to self-dosage of niacin, please remember that higher levels of niacin can be toxic, many possible drug interactions have to be considered, and there are several physical conditions (including pregnancy and lactation) with which niacin shouldn't be mixed. One might also discuss, with a pharmacist or physician, any complications which might result from the long term use of some types of slow-release niacin tablets.

One last note: In pellagra, the feces contain unusually large amounts of indole and skatole[21]. You will remember from chapter six that this is also true in schizophrenia.

Fig. 6. Locating the Pineal gland (discussed in Ch. 9.)

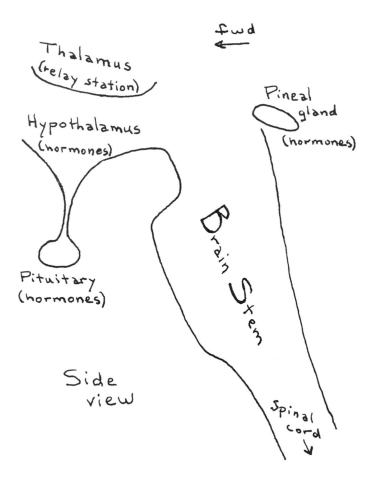

Ch 9

MELATONIN

Melatonin is another product of tryptophan which seems to be involved in a form of mental illness (Winter Depression-- S.A.D.--Seasonal Affective Disorder).

Melatonin is manufactured in the pineal gland (pineal body) of the brain (similar in appearance to the pituitary gland, but located opposite it--above the upper-rear of the brain stem, in an area actually considered outside the brain, since it's outside the blood-brain barrier), which takes tryptophan, makes it into serotonin, and that into melatonin. One of the results of my suggestions for bringing the blood tryptophan level up would be the availability of plenty of tryptophan to the pineal gland.

The pineal gland is thought to be involved in, among other things, the timing of when we wake in the morning, when we feel tired at night, when puberty and menopause start and when animals mate and migrate. The pineal gland is said to know day from night and winter from summer by the aid of offshoots from the optic nerves. These offshoots separate from the optic nerves at a place called the optic chiasm (the place where the optic nerves from the "inboard" sides of the two eyes cross over, allowing the right side of the brain to process what's seen by the right sides of both retinas, and the left side of the brain to handle what's seen by both left sides). Then the offshoots go to the pineal body, by way of a pair of nerve nuclei called the suprachiasmatic nucleus (which is in the hypothalamus, over the optic chiasm.). So, our pineals know when the sun comes up and when it goes down. By this, authorities tell us, it's able to time both the daily and seasonal functions of our bodies.

Melatonin is one of several hormones put out by the pineal gland. It was isolated around 1955 and found to be easily manufactured. Since then, progress in its study has been accelerating, especially in the last dozen years or so.

Melatonin has been found to be important to the body in several additional ways. Besides timing body functions, melatonin is thought to be a potent antioxidant and a scavenger of free radicals, and therefore is believed to act toward preventing cancer and to slow aging by preventing the destruction of cells. By destroying free radicals, melatonin may inhibit clotting in the coronary arteries. It has also been found to be active with the immune systems in several ways[1]. Melatonin may be important to the body in many other ways, but they aren't related to the subject of this book. There are several books available on melatonin.

It's said that the pineal gland makes serotonin continuously. If it also manufactures melatonin continuously, it stores the melatonin until sunset. When things are working as they should, the pineal puts out melatonin only at night. When evening darkness falls, the blood level of melatonin rises almost immediately, and when the sun rises in the morning, it drops almost immediately.

One might ask if melatonin is released when one enters

a dark room. The answer is no--the release is actually controlled by the suprachiasmatic nucleus (as mentioned above, a pair of nuclei in the hypothalamus), which is one of the body's internal clocks. It is regularly **reset** by sunrises and sunsets. (The clock feature of the neurons of the suprachiasmatic nucleus--the SCN--is amazing. If a single neuron is separated from an SCN and grown in culture, the cells of that culture still perform their various cell operations with a 24 hour rhythm.)[2]

That both the rising and the dropping of melatonin level should occur at the "proper" times seems to be important to the mental health of some people. **Seasonal affective disorder** is thought to occur because, in the far northern and southern latitudes in the wintertime, particularly near the arctic and antarctic circles, the sun comes up too late and goes down too early for the best timing of body functions. Melatonin production starts earlier in the evening and continues later into the morning than is best for the body. When a psychiatrist treats a person's **seasonal affective disorder** with a light box, he's causing that person's suprachiasmatic nucleus to reset its (morning) clock. (The light box puts out strong amounts of light at specific frequencies. Sitting at it for an hour (+ or -) on winter mornings, when the sun isn't yet up, is said to lead the pineal gland to "think" that the sun is up.)

Many people who don't live nearly as far north as the arctic circle suffer from seasonal affective disorder. On the other hand, not all of those who live in far-northern latitudes are bothered by it (it's estimated that 25 percent of those living in far-northern areas have the problem)[3].

Melatonin supplements are available, but these are best discussed with your physician.

Box 2. Derivation of Serotonin.

This is a little addition, only for those who are unbothered by long words. It does explain the derivation of 5-HTP, referred to in the next chapter.

1.) **Tryptophan**

(<u>enzyme</u>, tryptophan hydroxylase)

2.) **5-HTP** (5-OH-Tryp / 5-hydroxytryptophan)

(<u>enzyme</u>, 5-hydroxytryptophan decarboxylase)

3.) **Serotonin** (5HT / 5-hydroxytryptamine)

Ch 10

A LOOK TO THE FUTURE

Thank goodness, those who study mental illness have had an increasing interest in serotonin, because, to be interested in serotonin is really to be interested in tryptophan--and a lack of blood tryptophan is, in my opinion, the beginning of the depressive illnesses, schizophrenia and many other problems.

I hope that these concepts are accepted. The time has come for these illnesses to be cured. But while we wait for the realization of this hope...

I note that 5-HTP, the intermediate substance in the transformation of tryptophan to serotonin, has been prescribed with considerable success in other countries. In my opinion, if it isn't consumed by intestinal *E. coli*; and if it can pass readily from the intestine, to the blood, to the brain; and if it can reach neuron synapses to make serotonin, it may cure the depressive illnesses. If it can be used by the body to make niacin, it may prevent schizophrenia.

U.S. Health authorities haven't accepted 5-HTP

yet, because it's so closely related to tryptophan. They're still nervous, because of those tryptophan supplements that went wrong. We should check the results in Europe.

I'd also like to submit something relative to the treatment of bipolar (manic depressive) disorder. Bipolar depression affects at least one percent of the world's population. Happily, lithium compounds are able to help about eighty percent (eight out of ten) of those who suffer from this problem. Now, I'd like to make a suggestion that may help the other twenty percent (half-a-million people, in our country alone).

As is well known to chemists and pharmacists, lithium has two naturally ocurring isotopes (varieties) which occur mixed together in nature--Li6 and Li7--the one comprising about 7.5% and the other about 92.5% of the total. Although this is common knowledge, I find no mention of experiments on mental patients having been performed with carbonates of the separated isotopes.

Remembering the great differences between the uranium isotopes 235 and 238, which became extremely important in the search for atomic energy, I would suggest that the time has come for the two naturally occuring lithium isotopes to be separated and their carbonates tried, for their effectiveness in treating bipolar depression.

I hope that the separation and testing of the

lithium isotopes will soon be done, but I suspect that there will be a great dragging of feet, because of cost. Unless our government becomes involved, economics will make it a matter of comparing estimated cost of separating and testing against estimated income from sales, on the part of the pharmaceutical companies.

True, some pharmaceutical companies make large donations to worthy causes, but profit and loss usually have to be considered. Suffering doesn't have a column on profit and loss sheets and politicians may not even know the problem exists, unless the voice of the public is heard. Here is where **your** voice is needed, to your members of Congress. The lithium isotopes need to be separated and tested, so that **all** of those with bipolar disorder can (one hopes) be helped.

Now a few words about water pressure in the brain. Many years ago, I knew a gentleman named Ted, who had become ill with schizophrenia at about the age of thirty. He had been hospitalized, on and off, until they came out with the major tranquilizer drugs for schizophrenia, after which (when I knew him) he worked at menial jobs such as bus-boy in a restaurant (he was a truck driver, beforehand). When Ted was about sixty, he had more and more trouble walking. Finally, he couldn't even stand, unless held by two strong people (he was a big man).

His daughter took him to several doctors, determined to find out what was causing his walking and standing problems. All but one said that he had Parkinson's disease--and he did seem to make some progress on L-dopa. But his daughter was stubborn, and at last found one doctor who recognized the problem for what it was--a surgeon who realized that what Ted needed was a bypass-shunt operation, for excessive water pressure in the brain.

The day after the shunt operation, Ted was walking the hospital halls unaided, and soon he was walking so fast that I--a healthy 40 year-old who had done a lot of walking--could hardly keep up with him. (He retained his walking ability for the remaining fifteen years of his life.)

Ted's brother, who never had any mental problems, also had the shunt operation. Now approaching ninety, Ted's brother has as much trouble walking and standing as Ted used to have--and is being treated for Parkinson's.

I have several questions:

1) Considering the possible connection of serotonin with cerebrospinal fluid, were both Ted's schizophrenia and his water-pressure problems caused by a shortage of brain tryptophan and serotonin?

2) Could Ted's schizophrenia, which started long before the walking problem, have been aggravated by the early onset of the water-pressure problem? Is there any chance that excessive fluid pressure in the brain, as suggested in chapter eight, could be the cause of the enlarged ventricles (water-filled caverns

of the brain) found in schizophrenics--and if so, would all schizophrenics be helped by a shunt operation--or, by the proper amount of serotonin, which may be an inhibitor of the production of the fluid?

3) Are there any others, out there, being treated for Parkinson's disease, who really need a bypass-shunt operation?

4) What are the chances that Ted's brother's present problems (with walking and standing) are caused by a blockage of his bypass-shunt?

5) Are doctors who treat Parkinson's disease kept aware of the symptoms which call for a bypass-shunt operation, or indicate the blockage of a shunt already in place? Does anyone have the responsibility of reminding them?

6) Finally, would raising the brain serotonin level (by raising the brain tryptophan level) eliminate the need for such shunt operations?

Box 3. On needing <u>you</u>.

On this page, referring to the next chapter about the mentally ill needing <u>you</u>, I was tempted to place one of the old drawings of Uncle Sam, with his finger pointing at us--but with disheveled hair, a sad look and raggedy clothes. The subject of mental illness is too serious, however, for even something like that. We would all like to help these millions of people. But until now, the problem was to figure out what to do...

Ch 11

WHY THE MENTALLY ILL NEED YOU, THE READER

Following up on the ideas presented in this book may bring an end to much of the suffering of the mentally ill--and on the part of their relatives, as well. Nevertheless, we needn't expect those who work in the mental health field to quickly accept these ideas, and we needn't expect those who work in laboratories to rush to their labs to check them. That hasn't been the history of such things.

Sailing ships used to lose half their crews to scurvy. In 1564, a Dutch physician urged that sailors be fed citrus fruits to prevent scurvy (the Dutch were then very active on the seas). In 1639 (75 years later), a British doctor urged the same thing. A century later, a British naval doctor again urged the dietary change. But it was yet another sixty years before the British navy gave their crews citrus fruits[1] (frequently the juice of limes, perhaps in their rum), eliminated scurvy, and gave British sailors their nickname of Limeys.

In the industrial revolution in England (starting around 1760), children worked inside factories for double the number of hours that are now considered normal for adults in our country; they didn't get the sunshine that prevents rickets. So, while children were afflicted with bowed legs and curved spines, people laughed at the idea that these things could be caused by the lack of sunshine. Not until the 1800s was it learned that cod liver oil could replace the vitamin D that our skin manufactures in sunshine, and this concept wasn't well accepted until the 1900s.

In 1848, Dr. Theophile Roussel, a French doctor who was certain that a corn-only diet caused pellagra, was able to get his government to restrict the growing of corn--thus all but eliminating pellagra in France. But eighty years later, in the 1920s, 7000 people a year were still dying of pellagra in the United States, because of corn-only diets.[2] The American Indians, who gave us corn, didn't get pellagra because they ate other foods which gave them niacin and tryptophan, which prevent pellagra (you remember, the body makes supplemental niacin from tryptophan). The progress of pellagra was (as noted in chapter eight) dementia, dermatitis, diarrhea and death.

In the early 1880s, the Japanese navy recognized that the reason they were losing more than a thousand men a year from beriberi (over 6,000 men, in the years 1880-1883)[3] was that the polished rice they were feeding their sailors was lacking something; they eliminated beriberi by adding other foods to the sailor's diets. The finding wasn't accepted in the U.S. or Europe, because scientists here were looking for a bacterial cause for beriberi. Thousands continued to die of the disease in Southeast Asia (many of them in the Philippines, which was under our influence, at that time). It wasn't until 1920 that it was found that the rice polishings that were thrown away contained thiamine (vitamin B1).[4] The progress of beriberi was paralysis, dementia and death. (Since thiamine, among other things, helps to make niacin[5], that may account for the dementia.)

There are many other examples of our unwillingness to accept new ideas. Those in the health fields, feeling responsible for those whose lives are in their hands, have always been very careful in accepting new or different ideas. And in earlier times, communication of new ideas was very slow. If doctors didn't hear of new ideas, they could neither accept nor reject them.

Here again is where you, as a reader of this book, can help. The greater the number of doctors who read this book, the greater the chances are that these ideas will be accepted and acted upon. So, if you consider this book worthwhile and offer your book to a health professional to read and evaluate, **you may be the key to bringing about the cure of many mental illnesses.**

One final word. Before you or a loved one start any course of therapy for a mental problem--either a talking therapy or one with psychoactive drugs--**please** get a thorough physical examination and a thorough lab work-up. Many people who seem to be mentally ill, even to a psychiatrist, are really physically ill in some manner that produces the symptoms of mental illness. No form of therapy will detect this type of problem.

But the final words of this book should be about the book's main purpose. What this book is saying is that I don't think schizophrenia and the depressive illnesses are illnesses of the human body at all--but are the normal reactions of the body to a chronic shortage of tryptophan in the blood. I also suspect that the level of blood tryptophan which has heretofore been considered normal may in fact be a reduced level (reduced by the intestinal bacteria)--and that the brain of the average normal person is not receiving the optimal amount of tryptophan, and is not operating at its optimal level.

Please, therefore, join me in hoping that in another fifteen or twenty years, after a child is born, they'll put silver nitrate into its eyes and a small smear of the new *E. coli* bacteria at its anal area--and schizophrenia and depressive illness may join polio and smallpox in the past, and the mental level of the average normal person may be just a little higher (maybe, quite a bit higher) than it is now, and aggression may fade away.

In the meantime, if pyruvic acid capsules work out or if the needed *E. coli* bacterium is found or made, and soon used, those of us who are now alive may be healthier, happier and more mentally able, too.

GLOSSARY AND ABBREVIATIONS

5-HTP, the intermediate substance in the conversion of tryptophan to serotonin.

5-HT, serotonin.

5-HIAA, a breakdown product of serotonin, found in cerebrospinal fluid (which fills the ventricles of the brain and the areas around the spinal cord, and is eventually picked up by the blood).

ECT, electroconvulsive therapy, electrical shock treatment.

MAO, monoamine oxidase, the enzyme in neurons which breaks down serotonin and other chemical transmitters, after they are removed from the synapse.

MAOI, monoamine oxidase inhibitor, which inhibits the above MAO from breaking down serotonin and other transmitters.

MRI, magnetic resonance imaging.

NAD/NADH, substances produced by the body from niacin, active in mitochondria in the production of usable energy.

(Continued)

NADP/NADPH, substances produced by the body from NAD, active in the synthesis of important fatty acids, as well as necessary cholesterol.

Niacin, otherwise known as nicotinic acid; a B vitamin.

OCD, obsessive compulsive disease, a problem where the sufferer feels compelled to do repetetive actions.

Pyruvic acid, $CH_3COCOOH$. It's produced in cells by the breakdown of glucose.

SAD, winter depression or seasonal affective disorder, a mental problem of winter, apparently having to do with the hours of output of melatonin (see chapter 9).

SSRI, selective serotonin reuptake inhibitor, which inhibits the reuptake of serotonin from the synapse, thus increasing the amount of serotonin in the synapse.

Tryptophan, the amino acid (protein building block) from which, among other things, niacin, serotonin and melatonin are made, by the body.

Ventricles, the water-filled cavities of the brain.

BIBLIOGRAPHY

1) Aghajanian JK, Foote WE, Sheard MH: Action of psychotogenic drugs on midbrain raphe neurons. J Pharmacol Exp Ther 171, 1970.

2) Baldessarini R.J., Drugs and the treatment of psychiatric disorders, in The Pharmacological Basis of Theraputics, 4th Edition. Edited by Gilman A.G., Goodman I.S., Rall T.W., et al. New York, Macmillan, 1985.

3) Bear, Mark F., Ph.D., Barry W. Connors, Ph.D., and Michael A. Paradiso, Ph.D., Neuroscience: Exploring the Brain, published by Williams & Wilkins, a Waverly company, Baltimore, Maryland, 1996.

4) Bleich, A., Brown, S.L., Kahn, R., et al: The role of serotonin in schizophrenia. Schizophr. Bull. 14, 1988.

5) Cooper, Groffrey M., Ph.D., The Cell: A Molecular Approach, published by ASM Press, Washington, D.C.; Sinauer Associates, Inc., Sunderland, Massachusetts, 1997.

6) Devlin, Thomas M., Ph.D., Textbook of Biochemistry With Clinical Correlations, fourth edition, published by Wiley-Liss, Inc., 1997.

7) Dickinson, S.L., Curzon G.: Roles of dopamine and 5-hydroxy-tryptamine in steryotyped behavior. Nueropharmacology 22, 1983.

8) Glaser, T. and J.M. De Vry, Neurobiology of the 5HT$_{1A}$ Receptors, in Serotonin 1A Receptors, edited by Stahl, S.M., M. Gastpar, J.M. Kepper Hesselink and J. Traber, published by Raven Press, 1992, pp38,39.

9) Goldsmith, G.A., J. Amer. Diet. Assn. 32, 312 (1956).
From Eiduson, Samuel, Ph.D., Edward Geller, Ph.D.,
Arthur Yuwiler, Ph.D., Bernice T. Eiduson, Ph.D.,
Biochemistry and Behavior, published by D. Van Nost-
rand Company, Inc., Princeton, New Jersey, 1964, page 21,
(note 31).

10) Gorman, Jack M., M.D., The Essential Guide to Psychiatric
Drugs, published by St. Martin's Press, New York, 1990.

11) Jamison, Kay Redfield, Manic Depressive Illness and Creativity,
Scientific American, Feb. 1995.

12) Korsgaard S., Gerlach J., Christensson E.: Behavioral aspects of
serotonin-dopamine interaction in the monkey. Eur. Journal
of Pharmacology 118, 1985.

13) Kramer, Peter D., M.D., Listening To Prozac, published by
Viking Penguin, 1993, and Penguin Books, 1994.

14) Loudon, Marc G., Ph.D., Organic Chemistry, published by
The Benjamin/Cummings Publishing Company, Inc., 1995.

15) Mann, J. John, as reported from a 11/18/96 lecture on the neuro-
bilogy of suicide at the national meeting of the Society for
Neuroscience, Kansas City Star newspaper, pA-3,
Nov. 19, 1996.

16) Maxmen, Jerrold S., M.D., The New Psychiatry, published by
William Morrom and Co., Inc, N.Y., 1985.

17) Meltzer H.Y., Biological Studies in Schizophrenia.
Schiz. Bull. 13, 1987.

18) Miranda, Jeanne, Ann A. Hohmann, C. Clifford Attkisson and
David B.Larson, Editors, Mental Disorders in Primary
Care, published by Jossey-Bass Publishers, San Fransisco,
1994.

19) de Montigny, Claude, Pierre Blier, Electrophysiological Properties of 5-HT$_{1A}$ Receptors and of 5-HT$_{1A}$ Agonists, in Serotonin 1A Receptors, edited by Stahl, S.M., M. Gastpar, J.M. Kepper Hesselink and J. Traber, Published by Raven Press, 1992, pp86-87.

20) Ninan, P.T., Van Kammen, D.P., Scheinin, M., et al: CSF 5-hydroxyindole-acetic acid levels in suicidal schizophrenic patients, Am. J. Psychiatry 141, 1984.

21) Norden, Michael J., M.D., Beyond Prozac, published by Regan Books, an imprint of Harper Collins, Publishers, 1995.

22) Pierpaole, Walter, M.D., Ph.D. and William Regelson, M.D., The Melatonin Miracle, published by Simon and Schuster, 1995.

23) The Editors of **Prevention** Magazine, Understanding Vitamins and Minerals, published by Rodale Press, Emmaus, Pennsylvania, 1984.

24) Scala, James, Ph. D., Making the Vitamin Connection - The Food Supplement Story, published by Harper and Row, Publishers, New York, 1985.

25) Schatzberg, Alan F., M.D. and Charles B. Nemeroff, M.D., Ph.D., The American Psychiatric Press Textbook of Psychopharmacology, published by the American Psychiatric Press, Inc., Washington, D.C., London, England, 1995.

26) Shepherd, Michael, Editor, Psychiatrists on Psychiatry, published by Cambridge University Press, 1982.

27) Shepherd, Gordon M., M.D., D. Phil., Neurobiology (third edition), published by Oxford University Press, 1994.

28) Sourkes, Theodore L., Ph.D., Biochemistry of Mental Disease, published by Hoeber Medical Division, Harper and Row, 1962.

29) Tropp, Burton E., Professor, Dept. Of Chemistry and Biochemistry, Queens College, Biochemistry, Concepts and Applications, published by Brooks/Cole Publishing Company, 1997.

30) Wender, Paul H., M.D. and Donald F. Klein, M.D., Mind, Mood, and Medicine, published by McGraw-Hill Ryerson Ltd, Toronto, 1981.

31) Wild, Gaynor C. and Edward C. Benzel, Essentials of Neurochemistry, published by Jones and Bartlett, 1994.

32) Wurtman, Richard J. and Judith J. Wurtman, Carbohydrates and Depression, Scientific American, Jan. 1989.

33) Zeki, Semir, A Vision of the Brain, published by Blackwell Scientific Publications, London Edinburgh Boston Melbourne Paris Berlin Vienna, 1993.

34) Although I can't find the bacteriology book in which I first found this information, 30 or 35 years ago, the reference to indole and skatole is verified by Ref. 28, p79.

REFERENCES

Chapter 1
    1. Ref. 18, p4
    2. Ref. 30, p43
    3. Ref. 18, p4
    4. Ref. 18, pp20-21
    5. Ref. 16, pp15-16

Chapter 2
    1. Ref. 33, p183
    2. Ref. 3, p96

Chapter 4
    1. Ref. 11, pp62-63
    2. Ref. 11, p67
    3. Ref. 30, p23 and Ref. 11, p64
    4. Ref. 10, p204
    5. Ref. 11, p64
    6. Ref. 18, p7
    7. Ref. 18, p7

Chapter 5
    1. Ref. 10, p378
    2. Ref. 16, p215
    3. Ref. 26, p20
    4. Ref. 26, p187
    5. Ref. 25, p248
    6. Ref. 30, p146
    7. Ref. 30, p147
    8. Ref. 25, p248

Chapter 5 (continued)

9. Ref. 30, p23
10. Ref. 26, p193
11. Ref. 2, pp387-445
12. Ref. 25, p141
13. Ref. 25, p142
14. Ref. 13, p56
15. Ref. 13, pp60-64
16. Ref. 13, p66
17. Ref. 25, p789 and Ref. 21, p142
18. Ref. 25, p303
19. Ref. 25, p303
20. Ref. 16, pp126-127
21. Ref. 10, p158
22. Ref. 16, p116
23. Ref. 16, p161

Chapter 6
1. Ref. 34
2. Ref. 34
3. Ref. 32, p73

Chapter 7
1. Ref. 25, p51
2. Ref. 25, p170
3. Ref. 25, p57
4. Ref. 8, and Ref. 25, p53

Chapter 8
1. Ref. 15, pA-3
2. Ref. 31, pp67-69
3. Ref. 31, p68
4. Ref. 1, pp178-187

5. Ref. 19
6. Ref. 27, p558
7. Ref. 27, pp557-558
8. Ref. 21, p62
9. Ref. 12, pp245-252
10. Ref. 17, pp77-111
11. Ref. 20, pp566-569
12. Ref. 7, pp805-812 and Ref. 12, pp245-252
13. Ref. 4, pp297-315
14. Ref. 28, p223 and Ref. 24, p70
15. Ref. 28, p223
16. Ref. 9, p21
17. Ref. 14, p473
18. Ref. 29, p366
19. Ref. 5, p68
20. Ref. 6, p243
21. Ref. 28, pp79, 221

Chapter 9
1. Ref. 22, pp98-101
2. Ref. 3, pp480-482
3. Ref. 22, p197

Chapter 11
1. Ref. 23, p6
2. Ref. 23, p2
3. Ref. 23, p3
4. Ref. 23, pp4-5
5. Ref. 28, p223

INDEX

Order Form:

Please send me the book
Mental Illness For Caregivers.

Postal orders: Alma Publishing
                P.O. Box 28268
                Gladstone, MO 64188

Fax orders: (816) 459 4837

Tel. orders: (816) 459 9644 / (800) 997 4476

Online orders: almapubl@qni.com

Name:_____

Address:_____

City:_____State:_____Zip:_____

Telephone: (___)_____

Book Price: $9.95. (For multiple purchases, please
      call or write for discount and shipping.)

Shipping: Book rate (U.S. $), add $2.00 for U.S. or
      Canada; $2.25 for Mexico or foreign.
      First Class mail in U.S. $2.50.
      Priority Mail in U.S. $3.75.
      Air mail (U.S. $), Canada $2.40, Mex $2.60,
           foreign $7.75.

Sales Tax: For book shipped to **Missouri** address,
      please add $0.72 state tax.

Payment:

__Check

__Credit card: __MasterCard, __VISA,
      Other_____
      Card number: _____
      Name on card: _____
           Exp. date: ___/___

Order Form:

Please send me the book
Mental Illness For Caregivers.

Postal orders: Alma Publishing
P.O. Box 28268
Gladstone, MO 64188

Fax orders: (816) 459 4837

Tel. orders: (816) 459 9644 / (800) 997 4476

Online orders: almapubl@qni.com

Name:_____

Address:_____

City:_____State:_____Zip:_____

Telephone: (___)_____

Book Price: $9.95. (For multiple purchases, please
call or write for discount and shipping.)

Shipping: Book rate (U.S. $), add $2.00 for U.S. or
Canada; $2.25 for Mexico or foreign.
First Class mail in U.S. $2.50.
Priority Mail in U.S. $3.75.
Air mail (U.S. $), Canada $2.40, Mex $2.60,
foreign $7.75.

Sales Tax: For book shipped to **Missouri** address,
please add $0.72 state tax.

Payment:

__Check

__Credit card: __MasterCard, __VISA,
Other_____
Card number: _____
Name on card: _____
Exp. date: ___/___

Order Form:

Please send me the book
    Mental Illness For Caregivers.
Postal orders: Alma Publishing
                P.O. Box 28268
                Gladstone, MO 64188
Fax orders: (816) 459 4837
Tel. orders: (816) 459 9644 / (800) 997 4476
Online orders: almapubl@qni.com
Name:_____
Address:_____
City:_____State:_____Zip:_____
Telephone: (___)_____
Book Price: $9.95. (For multiple purchases, please
    call or write for discount and shipping.)
Shipping: Book rate (U.S. $), add $2.00 for U.S. or
    Canada; $2.25 for Mexico or foreign.
    First Class mail in U.S. $2.50.
    Priority Mail in U.S. $3.75.
    Air mail (U.S. $), Canada $2.40, Mex $2.60,
        foreign $7.75.
Sales Tax: For book shipped to **Missouri** address,
    please add $0.72 state tax.
Payment:
__Check
__Credit card: __MasterCard, __VISA,
    Other_____
    Card number: _____
    Name on card: _____
        Exp. date: ___/__